# THE EAT FIT COOKBOOK

## REVISED • UPDATED • EXPANDED

## CHEF INSPIRED RECIPES FOR THE HOME

### MOLLY KIMBALL
#### RD, LDN, CSSD

Photography by Emily Eickhoff, Teddie Taylor, and the Eat Fit Team

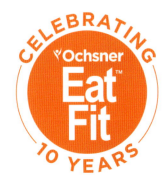

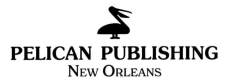

PELICAN PUBLISHING
NEW ORLEANS

Copyright © 2020, 2024
By Ochsner Clinic Foundation
All rights reserved

Front cover photograph by Sonia Savio
Front cover design by Cody Dingle
Back cover design by Matt Vermeulen

*Additional photography courtesy of:*

Tiffany McEntee (page 4)
Vieta Collins (page 6)
Marianna Massey (page 96)
Chris Granger (page 103)
WYES-TV Good Eating...Good Health (page 160)
and Mike Hartnet (page 206)

First River Road Press edition, 2020
First Pelican edition, 2024

*The word "Pelican" and the depiction of a pelican are trademarks of Arcadia Publishing Company Inc. and are registered in the U.S. Patent and Trademark Office.*

ISBN: 9781455626281

Printed in China
Published by Pelican Publishing
New Orleans, LA
www.pelicanpub.com

# Contents

**FOREWORD** — 5

**ACKNOWLEDGMENTS** — 7

**THE EAT FIT STORY** — 10

**1 SHARE** / Starters + Small Bites — 15

**2 BOWLS** / Bisques, Soups + Spoonables — 47

**3 CRISP** / Starter Salads, Fruits + Foliage — 79

**4 MAIN** / Entrées + Entrée Salads — 97

**5 LAGNIAPPE** / Accompaniments + Sides — 149

**6 DRIZZLE** / Dressings, Vinaigrettes + Sauces — 169

**7 INDULGE** / Sweets, Treats + Bakery — 189

**8 SIP** / Cocktails, Zero Proof Cocktails + Refreshers — 217

**INDEX** — 239

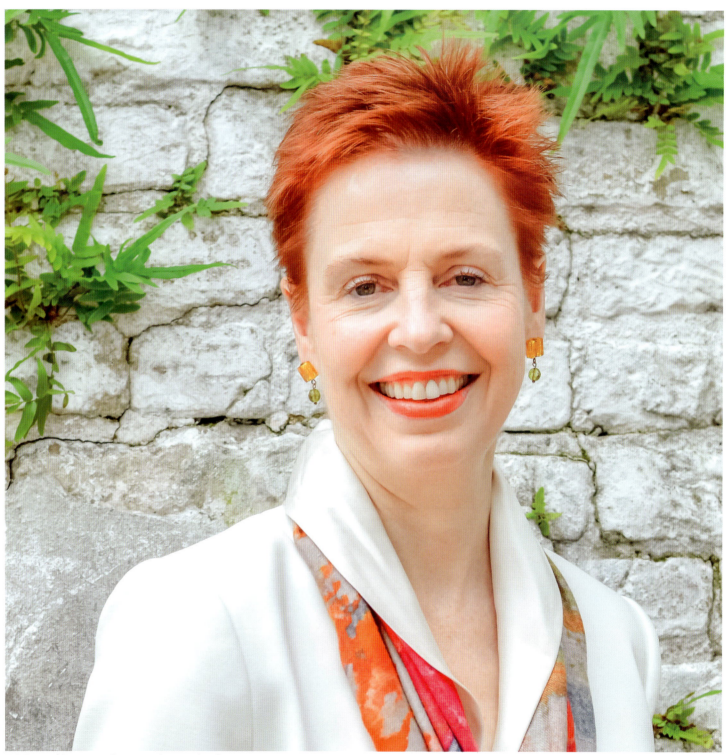

Ti Martin (Courtesy Commander's Palace)

# Foreword

In the 1990s Commander's Palace started providing what we called "Heart Healthy" menu options at lunch. We were inspired by the "heart attack pack," whose members included my mother Ella Brennan-Martin, her two brothers John and Dick, and John's wife Claire, who had all had heart surgery within a couple of years of each other. And we had very regular guests—at lunch, in particular—who wanted to "behave a little." So we started working with Ochsner to give us guidelines and check our recipes a bit.

Not too long into that process we met one Molly Kimball. Well, what a journey we embarked on with Molly.

Something became clear very quickly: Molly was on a mission. No amount of foot-dragging or excuses about busy brunches or flirting by the sous chef and cooks who thought she was adorable would slow her up. Molly was convinced we could create great-tasting dishes that fit her stringent guidelines.

She pushed, smiled, and pushed some more. She gave us substitute ingredient ideas, and she checked and measured and checked and measured. She put up with no shenanigans. If the recipes looked iffy to her or the execution she enjoyed in the dining room didn't seem to be quite the same as the one she approved, I would get the phone call: "Ti, I love you guys but . . ." The chefs learned quickly, and over the years, we have created literally hundreds of Eat Fit dishes.

All this time Molly has been talking about these dishes during her TV appearances and in her newspaper column. She is making New Orleans think about eating healthier. Now THAT is an accomplishment.

Then she calls one day. "Ti, what do you think about us expanding Eat Fit NOLA to other restaurants in New Orleans?" Well, we loved the idea. Secretly though, knowing the resistance of some of our cooks, I knew how hard this would be.

And off she went. No overnight success. Just hard work—blocking and tackling, we call it. She cold-called chefs and restaurateurs, she cajoled, she charmed, whatever it took. Well, it's all over New Orleans now and other cities are launching the program. How about that!

The truth is, Eat Fit is as much a part of New Orleans now as fried catfish (sorry about the fried, Molly) on Fridays during Lent. It will be with us forever. New Orleans loves it.

And truth be told, to change the eating culture of New Orleans and beyond—just a little—is one heck of an accomplishment.

Molly, we thank you and we love you.

—*Ti Adelaide Martin*
*and the Commander's Palace family*

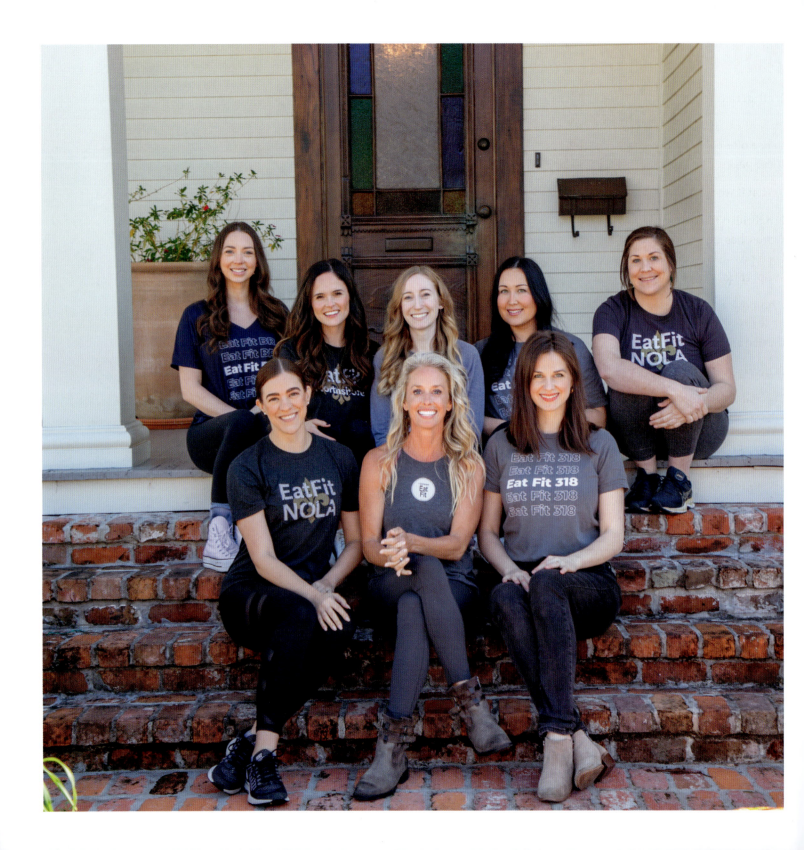

# Acknowledgments

It all started with "What if . . ."

Two of my favorite words. Two words I encourage our team to use often. The two words that are the reason you're reading these pages.

"What if we created an Eat Fit cookbook?"

I'm thrilled that the seed of an idea that started with these two words has become reality. And this reality would not have been possible without the passion, teamwork, dedication, and support from so many.

And now, for this revised and expanded second edition—and as we celebrate the 10-year anniversary of Ochsner Eat Fit—this list is even bigger.

A tremendous thank you to:

The Eat Fit chefs, restaurants, markets, and product partners who generously shared their recipes for this cookbook.

Emily Eickhoff, longtime Eat Fit ambassador who dove headfirst into this project as researcher, project manager, and photographer for the first edition of the Eat Fit Cookbook.

Savanna Latimer, Eat Fit Baton Rouge registered dietitian and project manager for this second edition of the Eat Fit Cookbook.

Hope Frugé, Eat Fit Monroe registered dietitian and photography director for this second edition of the Eat Fit Cookbook.

The rest of our Eat Fit team, who worked with their region's culinary partners to bring these new recipes to life. They photographed the beautiful dishes, edited recipe copy, and put recipes to the test in their own kitchens: Brittany Craft, Emma Poling, Annie Kent, Anna White, and Erin Arceneaux.

The Eat Fit and Ochsner Fitness Center Nutrition teams past and present, who contributed to the first edition: Brittany Craft, Savanna Latimer, Alexis Weilbaecher Thompson, Rebecca Miller, Lauren Hulin Berry, Yvette Perrier Quantz, Vanessa Richard, and Jala Lockhart. Thank you for your input, support, recipe analysis, and quadruple-checking nutrition facts and claims.

The many, many Eat Fit ambassadors over the years. Eat Fit would not be what it is today without you.

Diedra Dias, for believing in Eat Fit, seeing the potential for what it could be, and your support in making this a reality.

Matt Vermeulen for (again) so generously sharing your time, talents, and expertise in the cover design and the look and feel of the pages throughout.

The talented photographer Sonia Savio—thank you for your perseverance to capture the cover photo. And to photographer Teddie Taylor; we love you and appreciate the abundance of beauty you created within these pages. Your photographs of Chef Leah Chase are among my favorites.

The cookbook advisory panel of Ti Martin and Alexis Korman. Thank you for so generously sharing your expertise and wisdom. And an additional thank you to Ti for believing in me and my mission with Eat Fit in restaurants long before anyone else.

To Ben McLauchlin, Andress Blackwell, and Amy Davis for sharing your deliciously sweet recipes, expertise, and positivity with us.

The recipe testers: family, friends, interns, coworkers, and some people we've never met but who so graciously offered to help. Your experience and feedback were invaluable.

The Foodcare team, Ken Marshall and Lisa Luong, the brains and expertise behind our Eat Fit mobile app.

The leadership team at Ochsner Health, past and present, and our Ochsner Fitness Center family. Thank you for believing in us and in this project and for your support to do what we love.

The Pelican Publishing team for executing our vision, including publisher Scott Campbell, editor-in-chief Nina Kooij, and senior production manager Julie Buckner.

And finally, I am so grateful for the support, love, and enthusiasm of my husband, Brad. Everything is better, brighter, and funnier with you.

# A Special Thank You

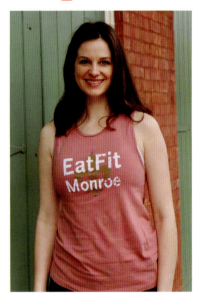

**Hope Frugé, Photography Director**

Hope's official title with our team is Eat Fit Monroe registered dietitian. But lucky us, Hope also brings with her a strong background in communications and photography—including a stint as *Edible Nashville*'s associate editor—positioning her perfectly to provide creative direction and image editing for this project.

Recognized as Miss Louisiana 2011, a Top 20 Under 40 business professional, and awarded the Women's Symposium's 2017 Rising Young Professional Award, Hope was also the sole photographer for our second book, *Craft: The Eat Fit Guide to Zero Proof Cocktails*.

But, above all else, her favorite thing is to simply be anywhere with her husband, Heath, and their daughters, Landry and Marienne.

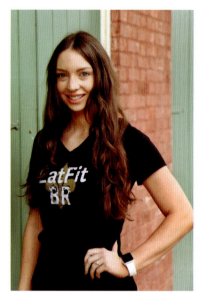

**Savanna Latimer, Project Manager**

Our Eat Fit Baton Rouge registered dietitian and project manager for this edition of The Eat Fit Cookbook, Savanna also led our team throughout the creation of our second book, *Craft: The Eat Fit Guide to Zero Proof Cocktails*. From recipe analysis and editing to proofreading and coordinating recipe testers, Savanna's organizational skills and attention to detail keep us focused and on task.

When she is not working with Eat Fit or teaching group fitness classes, Savanna enjoys spending time with her family, traveling, and long walks with her husband Dustin, daughter Roe, and her golden retriever Stella.

### Eat Fit Cookbook Recipe Testers

A tremendous thank you to our recipe testers who generously and enthusiastically volunteered their time and talents:

**2019 Edition**

Andre Burvant • Julie Bonano • Allyson Cabes • Cheryl Cabes • Jill Cabes • Lorie Demarcay • Diedra Dias • Rob Dille • Tod Everedge • Ann De Montluzin Farmer • Ashley Ferdinand • Pat Kimball • Kim Kringlie • Kristina Larson • Jala Lockhart • Ann Maloney • Stephanie Myers • Yvette Quantz • Vanessa Richard • Brad Schlotterer • Carolyn Schlotterer • Lindsey Schlotterer • Peggy Schlotterer • Tracey Schlotterer • Nell Simpson • Katie Jo Styczynsi • Leah Talbot • Linda Teen • Noel Teen Simmons • Dylan Thriffiley • Nicole Waguespack

**2023 Edition**

Jessica Bach • Matt Farah • Suzy Faucheux • Mary Beth Fishback • Cyndi Hanford • Carla Ingle • Annie Kent • Susan Lynd • Grace Mobley • Thomas K. Nguyen • Carla Pittari • Lydia Ratliff • Emerson Riley • Sarah Riley • Patricia Ross • Allie Segura • Becky Spinnato • Matt Standefer • Sarah Standefer • Rachael Swanson • Nathan Tipton • Anna White • Kay White • Amanda Wildblood

# About Molly

As the founder of Ochsner Eat Fit, registered dietitian Molly Kimball's approachable wellness philosophy has influenced the lives of thousands.

Molly and her team of Eat Fit dietitians work with hundreds of restaurant partners across Louisiana to develop and identify nutritious items on the menu with the mission of providing easy-to-access real-world wellness education, inspiration, and resources.

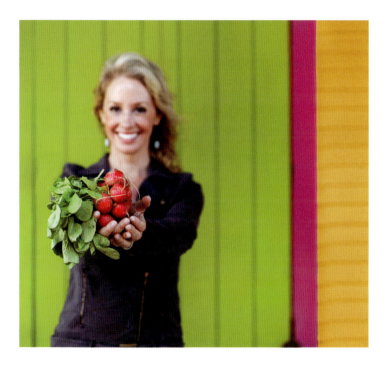

Board certified as a specialist in sports dietetics by the Academy of Nutrition and Dietetics, Molly is the director of nutrition at Ochsner Fitness Center where she leads the Lifestyle Nutrition team of dietitians as they guide clients in achieving and exceeding their wellness goals.

A nutrition journalist, Molly covers all things related to wellness and nutrition. She served as nutrition columnist for the *Times-Picayune* from 2009-19 and has been the nutrition expert for New Orleans' ABC affiliate WGNO since 2009, with weekly TV segments on *Good Morning New Orleans*, "FUELED Wellness + Nutrition with Molly." Molly also hosts a weekly podcast of the same name, "FUELED Wellness + Nutrition."

*The Eat Fit Cookbook* is Molly's first book. Her second, *Craft: The Eat Fit Guide to Zero Proof Cocktails* (Pelican Publishing, 2022) features more than fifty Eat Fit, zero proof drink recipes as well as guides to barware, bitters, glassware, and everything needed to create a fully sensorial cocktail.

Molly prefers a good walk-and-talk with colleagues versus desk or video meetings, and when she's not immersed in the world of nutrition science, you can find her creating functional pottery, a perfect antidote to technology and deadlines.

# The Eat Fit Story

The Crescent City is well known for its reputation of debauchery and divine, deep-fried delicacies. In our culture, food is more than nutrition—it's an obsession. Five minutes after lunch, we're talking about dinner. But usually we are talking about the decadence of our meals, not the healthfulness.

We love dining out, and New Orleans is one of the best places in the world to do so. However, as a registered dietitian and nutrition journalist in the New Orleans area for more than 20 years, it hasn't always been so easy to find nutritious options at our famous restaurants.

So, we collaborated with some of the most iconic restaurants in the New Orleans area to create Ochsner Eat Fit, a nonprofit initiative that encourages chefs to offer nutritious, delicious menu options for those who want to eat clean, look better, and feel better, and also for those watching their weight, blood sugar, blood pressure, and cholesterol. Our goal is to take the guesswork out of dining healthfully, making the healthy choice the easy choice.

And, it's working!

Today, Eat Fit recipes are featured in more than 600 restaurants across the state, including Commander's Palace, Ye Olde College Inn, and Mosca's. Eat Fit can be found in the area's largest tourist destinations, such as the Superdome, Jazz Fest, and the Louis Armstrong New Orleans International Airport. Eat Fit approved items are on the menu at local schools, and we are beyond thrilled that, each Carnival season, our Eat Fit king cake is available in retailers across the states of Louisiana and Texas.

As our beloved friend and Eat Fit Chef Ambassador Carl Schaubhut used to say, "If you can make this work in New Orleans, you can do it anywhere!"

Our Eat Fit cookbook shares our restaurant partners' delicious recipes and arms home cooks with tips and tricks they can use in their own kitchens, at the grocery store, and in their daily meal presentations to amp up their dinner game. We also provide insight and share tips of the nutrition trade to help you make better choices in your daily food decisions, not just when preparing these dishes.

There's a lot of misinformation and misperception about what we should and shouldn't eat. We cut through this confusion and teach readers how to optimally fuel their bodies with foods they love. We've included educational features, charts, and visuals to answer some of the most common questions we hear in our work as registered dietitians. Our goal is to make it easy to nourish our bodies, look and feel great, and live our strongest, healthiest lives possible.

## How Eat Fit Started

When I am dining out, it's not uncommon to run into clients, readers, and viewers who turn to me for guidance in the sometimes-daunting task of navigating a restaurant menu, seeking out the better-for-you fare. People often want to make the healthy choice, but they don't know how.

My husband suggested I do something about it—work with restaurants to incorporate nutritious options onto their menus. But where would I even begin?

Enter Ochsner Health, my employer of more than 20 years. Our then-CEO, Dr. Patrick Quinlan, wanted Ochsner to have a bigger and broader impact on the communities it served. He asked me how we might reach people before they became our patients.

Roughly half of American adults have at least one chronic health condition such as heart disease, cancer, diabetes, obesity, or arthritis. The good news is that science continues to show us that we can prevent or manage nearly all of these through nutrition and lifestyle changes. Combine this with the fact that nearly half of our food dollars are spent away from the home, and the answer to Dr. Quinlan's question was remarkably clear.

I proposed to Ochsner a program that married the two: work

with local restaurants to incorporate nutritious-yet-still-delicious items onto the menu, eliminating the guesswork for consumers who want to dine healthfully.

We were already working with Commander's Palace, a New Orleans culinary landmark, to highlight heart-healthy choices on their menu. I wanted to take it a few nutritional steps further, and if one chef was willing to do it, perhaps I could get more to join.

Eat Fit, a nonprofit initiative of Ochsner Health, was born in 2013.

## How Eat Fit Works

Our approach is straightforward: our team of dietitians works closely with restaurants, markets and other food service establishments to identify and develop dishes that meet the Eat Fit nutritional criteria. These items are highlighted directly on the restaurant's menu with the Eat Fit seal. (And it's no surprise that every recipe in this book has the Eat Fit seal of approval!)

The Eat Fit nutritional criteria are centered on foods and nutrients that help us look and feel our best. They're also designed with a preventive and therapeutic approach in mind. No refined carbohydrates, a lighter hand on salt, little or no added sugar, and a greater emphasis on plant-based fats means that Eat Fit is a perfect choice for those watching their waistlines, as well as blood sugar, blood pressure, and cholesterol levels. Eat Fit dishes are also naturally rich in anti-inflammatory compounds, linked to a host of benefits from our mood to our joints to our hearts. Basically, more of the stuff we want in our foods, and less (or none) of the stuff we don't want (for full details on Eat Fit nutritional criteria, visit OchsnerEatFit.org).

Originally when we approached restaurants with the Eat Fit concept, some thought we were a little nuts. "Guests want to indulge, not watch their waistlines," chefs said. "A slimmed-down version of shrimp and grits won't taste good." But ultimately, top New Orleans chefs gave us the opportunity to prove that there is a market for healthier options—not only for the 10 million tourists who dine at our acclaimed restaurants each year, but also for our residents who live and work in New Orleans.

We dove into menus to find dishes that needed just a slight tweak or two to become Eat Fit-approved. In some cases, we collaborated with chefs to create entirely new dishes.

We refuse to change the fabric of the great dishes that our chefs create, and we don't want our recipe edits to be noticeable to their guests. An Eat Fit dish has to make the chef proud and pass the customer taste test.

The recipes found throughout our cookbook are home versions of these dishes that our chefs created for Eat Fit. All have appeared on restaurant menus across the state or have been featured on various media outlets. All have been tested in home kitchens for ease of preparation.

Through Eat Fit, we've connected with our community of chefs in ways that we never expected, gently guiding and encouraging subtle lifestyle changes that impact not just their menus, but also the wellness of the chef, their staff, and their families.

By using these recipes and trying the suggested tips and techniques, you will learn how to transform your favorite recipes and expand your repertoire far beyond the recipes in this book. We can't dine out all the time—but there's no reason the food we eat at home can't taste like it was made by a famous chef. The recipes in this book will eliminate the nutrition guesswork and help all of us Eat Fit any time, any place.

## The Eat Fit Team

As we celebrate the 10-year anniversary of Ochsner Eat Fit, one of the things that I am most proud of is our strong and cohesive team of dietitians across the state. They are loving, hardworking, and beautifully supportive of one another as they continue to grow as leaders and role models within their communities, spreading the Eat Fit message within their own regions.

# Pantry

Here's your snapshot of what we keep in the kitchen at all times. Stock your kitchen with the essentials to whip up Eat Fit goodness any time.

## Fridge
- Low fat (2%) plain Greek yogurt
- Unsweetened vanilla almond milk
- Eggs
- Goat Cheese
- Berries (any variety)
- Coffee concentrate
- Flavored sparkling water

## Dry Goods
- Almond flour
- Coconut flour
- Xanthan gum
- Swerve Granular
- Swerve Confectioners
- Swerve Brown Sugar Replacer
- Cocoa powder
- Cacao
- Vanilla extract
- Canned unsweetened coconut milk
- Unsalted broth or stock (chicken or vegetable)

## Herbs + Spices
- Fresh ginger root
- Minced garlic
- Tabasco
- Sea salt
- Black peppercorn (plus grinder)

## Oils + Vinegars
- Extra virgin olive oil
- Light olive oil
- Avocado oil
- Coconut oil
- Nonstick cooking spray
- Apple cider vinegar
- Balsamic vinegar

## Supplements
- Collagen powder
- Vanilla protein powder

# Kitchen Tools

We're not big on gadgets that just clutter things up. But we're crazy about kitchen tools that we actually use, especially those that save us oodles of time. Here are 6 kitchen basics that we use all the time. If you don't have these on hand already, consider adding them to your kitchen essentials. We promise you won't regret it.

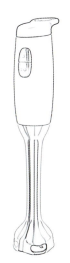

**Immersion Blender:** Makes it easier than ever to blend ingredients directly in the pots you're cooking with or the bowls they are served in; perfect for sauces and soups.

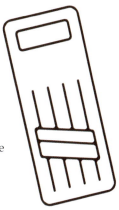

**Mandoline:** Shave and slice foods into incredibly thin, consistent pieces. Most also come with attachments for julienne style and crinkle cuts.

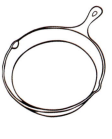

**Cast-Iron Skillet:** It's one of the few kitchen tools that gets better with age. Over time, it essentially becomes a nonstick pan that's practically indestructible. To clean, wash it under running water with little or no soap (for deeper cleaning, scrub with a paste of coarse salt and water) and wipe dry. Rub with a very light layer of oil and store in a dry place.

**Parchment Paper:** It's versatile, perfect for lining baking sheets or to make cleanup easy. Be aware, though, that parchment and wax paper are not the same thing. Parchment paper can take the heat of the oven, while wax paper cannot; if heated, the wax could melt or even catch on fire. Nobody wants that.

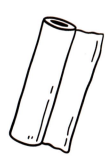

**Prep Bowls + Ramekins:** These little stackable bowls make prep work easy—and pretty—if you're into snapping photos for social media while you cook.

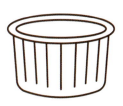

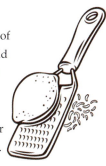

**Microplane:** Think of it as a mini handheld cheese grater, ideal for zesting fruit, grating garlic, or shredding butter (or cheese) into recipes.

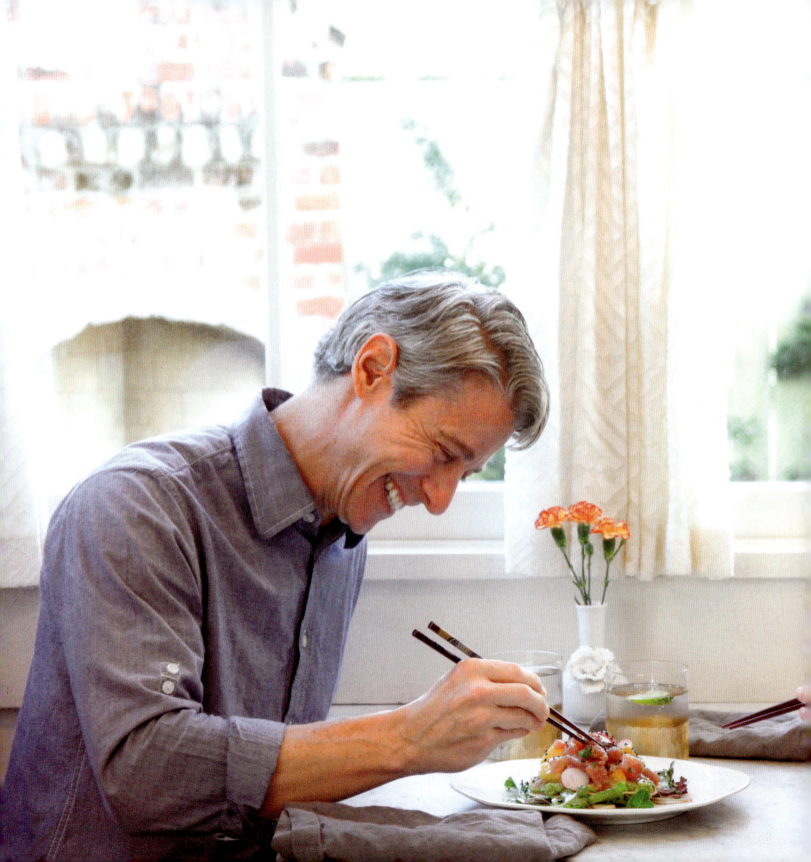

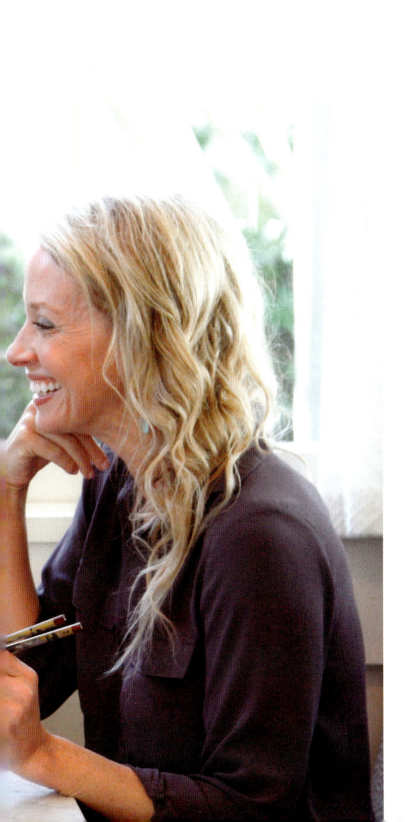

# 1
# SHARE
## Starters + Small Bites

Let's be honest, no one wants to be "that person"—the one who shows up to parties with a raw veggie platter in tow. While it may appeal to fellow health-conscious friends, it just doesn't pack an enticing punch next to sauced-up, fried-up favorites.

Eat Fit bites, snacks, and appetizers are a fabulous opportunity to introduce friends and family to delicious yet nutritious options. These dishes are beautiful, decadent and—best of all—Eat Fit approved. We serve and share these at tailgates with friends, on family beach vacations, and at home for any and all occasions. And trust me, they're always a hit.

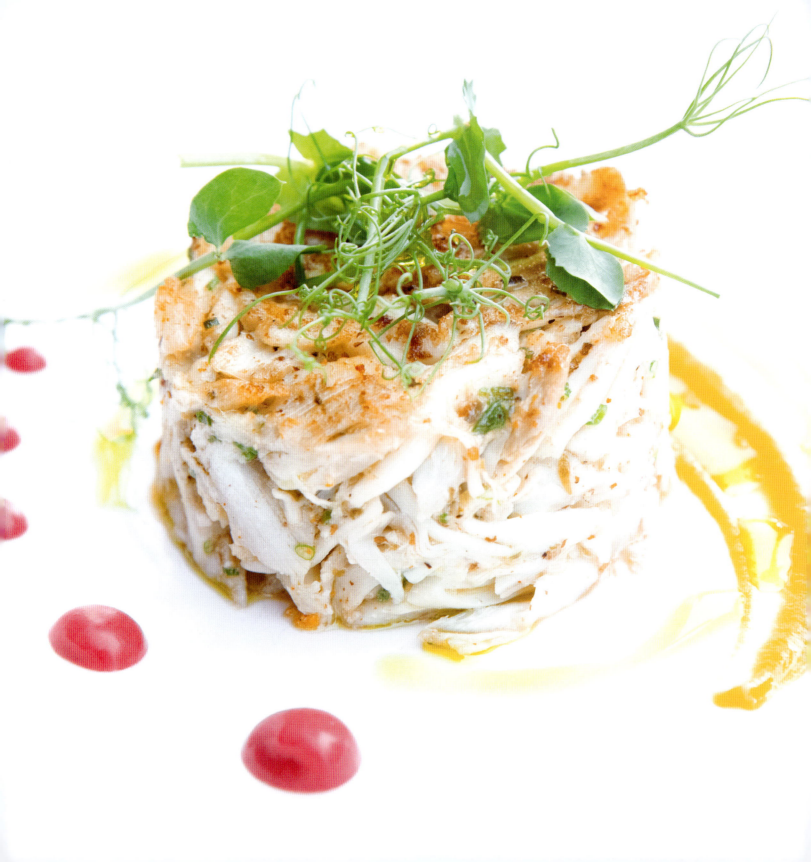

# Jumbo Lump Crab Cakes
## *Dickie Brennan's Steakhouse*

**Makes 8 servings**

Crazy-low in carbs, these divine crab cakes contain zero breadcrumbs or fillers and pair well with just about any grilled or sautéed vegetable. Our favorite accompaniments are grilled asparagus or creamy whipped cauliflower. Prepare in half-portions or minis for a distinctive, pre-dinner "shareable."

**2 pounds jumbo lump crabmeat**
**¼ cup chopped fresh parsley**
**6 ounces Ravigote Sauce (page 183)**
**½ red onion, diced**
**½ small red pepper, diced**
**¼ teaspoon freshly ground black pepper**

In a large mixing bowl, combine all ingredients, tossing until evenly mixed. Place approximately ½ cup of the crab mixture into a 3-inch ring mold. Heat skillet to medium-high heat and cook the crab cake—still inside the mold—until seared and golden brown on top and bottom. Serve immediately.

**PER SERVING:** 150 calories, 5 grams fat, 0.5 grams saturated fat, 500 mg sodium, 2 grams carbohydrate (2 grams net carbs), 0 fiber, <1 gram sugar (0 added sugar), 23 grams protein
**GF, Low Carb**

## Sodium Check

The sodium is a smidge (okay, 100 mg) higher than Eat Fit criteria for an appetizer. But we let this slide since this dish has enough protein to also serve as an entrée.

Crabmeat is naturally high in sodium, contributing more than 60% of the sodium in this dish, so it's tough to create a truly low-sodium crab cake. If you're looking to keep sodium really tight, make mini crab cakes using a smaller ring mold.

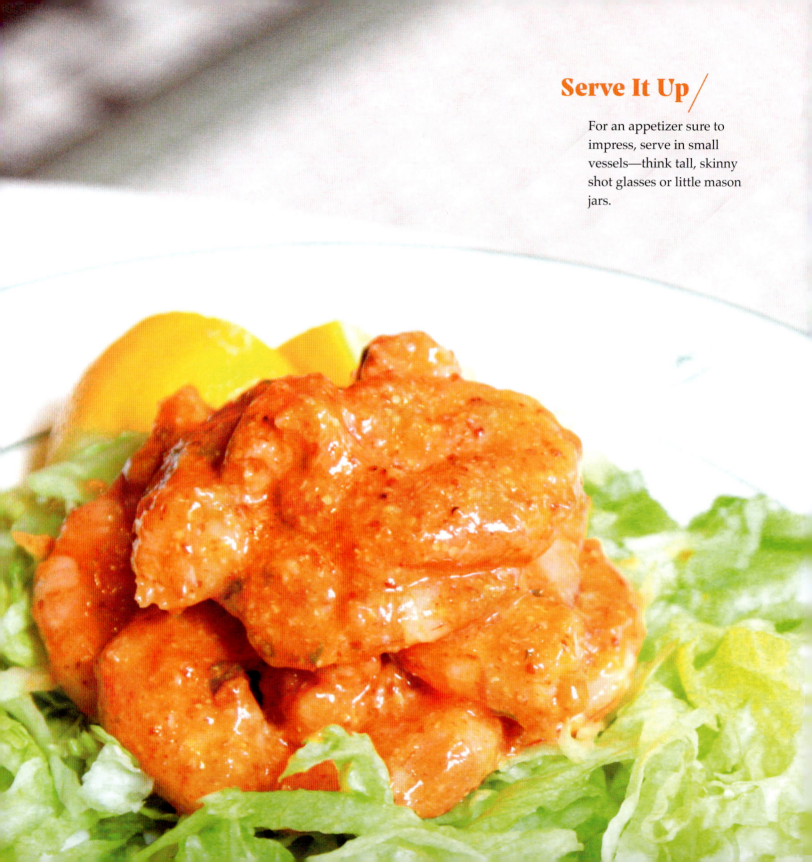

### Serve It Up

For an appetizer sure to impress, serve in small vessels—think tall, skinny shot glasses or little mason jars.

# Shrimp Remoulade
## Galatoire's

**Makes 8 servings**

Will wonders never cease? Yes, this iconic Galatoire's recipe qualifies as an Eat Fit approved dish! Elegantly nestled along Bourbon Street in the French Quarter, Galatoire's is not only one of New Orleans' finest restaurants, it is also a paragon of tradition.

**2 cups Remoulade Sauce (page 181)**
**2 pounds jumbo shrimp (approximately 4 dozen shrimp), peeled, boiled, and chilled**
**1 small head of iceberg lettuce, washed, dried, and sliced into thin ribbons**
**2 lemons, cut into wedges**

In a large mixing bowl, add Remoulade Sauce to shrimp and toss gently to coat. Divide lettuce among 8 chilled salad plates. Divide shrimp evenly atop the lettuce, garnish with lemon wedge, and serve.

**PER SERVING:** 190 calories, 7 grams fat, 1 gram saturated fat, 360 mg sodium, 6 grams carbohydrate (5 grams net carbs), 1 gram fiber, 3 grams sugar (0 added sugar), 24 grams protein
**GF, Low Carb**

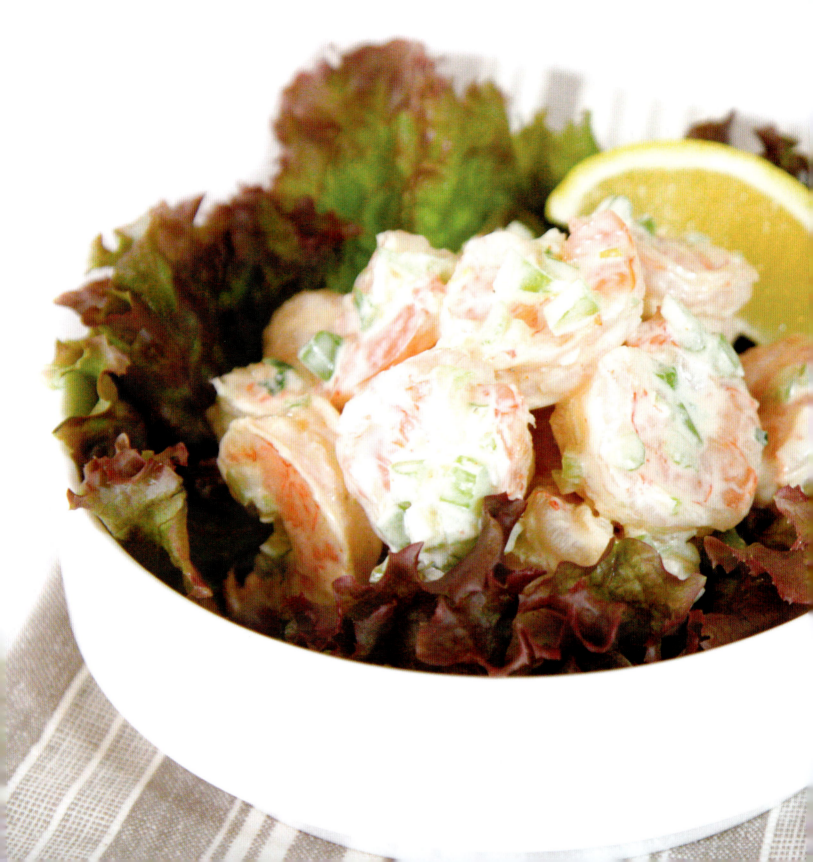

# Shrimp Salad with Raspberry Mint Vinaigrette
## Caffe! Caffe!

**Makes 6 servings**

Creamy doesn't have to mean unhealthy, and Caffe! Caffe! proves it with one of its most popular menu items. This neighborhood favorite features a heaping scoop of shrimp salad that boasts less than 200 calories and a mere 6 grams of carbs.

1¼ pounds medium shrimp, boiled and cleaned
¾ cup diced celery
½ tablespoon diced green onion
¼ teaspoon sea salt
¼ teaspoon freshly ground black pepper
¼ teaspoon cayenne
⅓ cup mayonnaise
6 hearts romaine lettuce or curly lettuce leaves
6 tablespoons Raspberry Mint Vinaigrette (page 177)
1 lemon, cut into wedges

In a large bowl, combine shrimp, celery, green onion, salt, pepper, and cayenne. Add mayonnaise and mix thoroughly.

Serve as single-serving "cups" inside of hearts of romaine lettuce or curly lettuce leaves, each drizzled with 1 tablespoon of Raspberry Mint Vinaigrette and a lemon wedge for garnish.

**PER SERVING:** 190 calories, 9 grams fat, 1.5 gram saturated fat, 220 mg sodium, 6 grams carbohydrate (6 grams net carbs), 0 fiber, 3 grams sugar (0 added sugar), 23 grams protein
GF, Low Carb

**Tip**

Turn it into a taco or lettuce wrap.

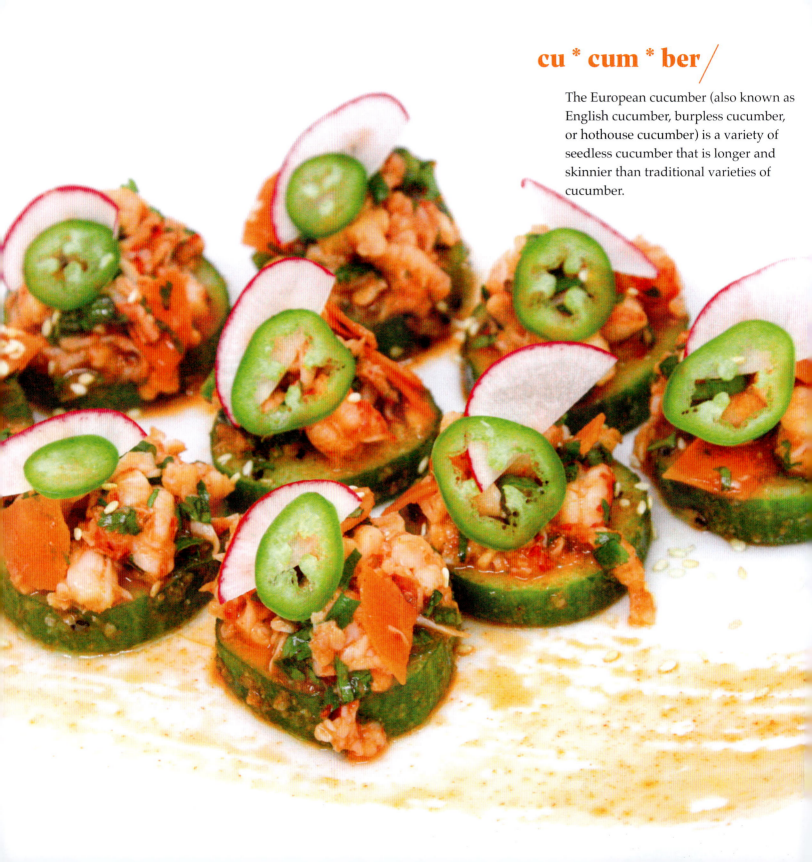

# cu * cum * ber /

The European cucumber (also known as English cucumber, burpless cucumber, or hothouse cucumber) is a variety of seedless cucumber that is longer and skinnier than traditional varieties of cucumber.

# Vietnamese-Style Crawfish Canapé on Spiced Cucumber Medallions

*Chef Carl Schaubhut*

**Makes 8 servings**

Lovely, fresh, and light, Chef Carl's mouthwatering Spiced Cucumber Medallions are naturally low in carbs.

**For the Crawfish**
- 1 pound Louisiana crawfish tails, rinsed and pressed gently to dry
- ¼ cup Miso Vinaigrette (page 171)
- 1 teaspoon Chinese Five Spice
- 2 tablespoons hot sauce
- 1 teaspoon fish sauce

**For the Canapé**
- 1 carrot, grated into matchsticks
- ½ cup chopped fresh cilantro
- ½ cup green onions, julienned
- 2 European cucumbers, cut into ¼-inch rounds
- 1 tablespoon sesame oil
- 2 tablespoons sesame seeds, divided
- ¼ cup shaved radish for garnish
- 1 jalapeño, shaved

**Prepare the Crawfish:** Preheat oven to 400 degrees. Toss crawfish tails with Miso Vinaigrette, Chinese Five Spice, hot sauce, and fish sauce. Spread onto a baking sheet and roast for 5 minutes. Remove from heat and refrigerate for at least 1 hour or until chilled.

**Assemble the Canapé:** In a large mixing bowl, combine crawfish, carrot, cilantro, and green onions and set aside.

Toss cucumbers with sesame oil and 1 tablespoon sesame seeds. Top cucumber slices with crawfish mix. Garnish with remaining sesame seeds, shaved radish, and shaved jalapeño.

**PER SERVING:** 170 calories, 12 grams fat, 1.5 grams saturated fat, 210 mg sodium, 6 grams carbohydrate (5 grams net carbs), 1 gram fiber, 3 grams sugar (0 added sugar), 11 grams protein

LOW CARB

## Time Saver

Make the crawfish ahead of time so all you have to do is cut the cucumber and you'll be ready to serve.

## Kick It Up

Chinese Five Spice—a blend of cinnamon, cloves, fennel, star anise, and Szechwan peppercorns—is easy to make or readily available at Asian markets.

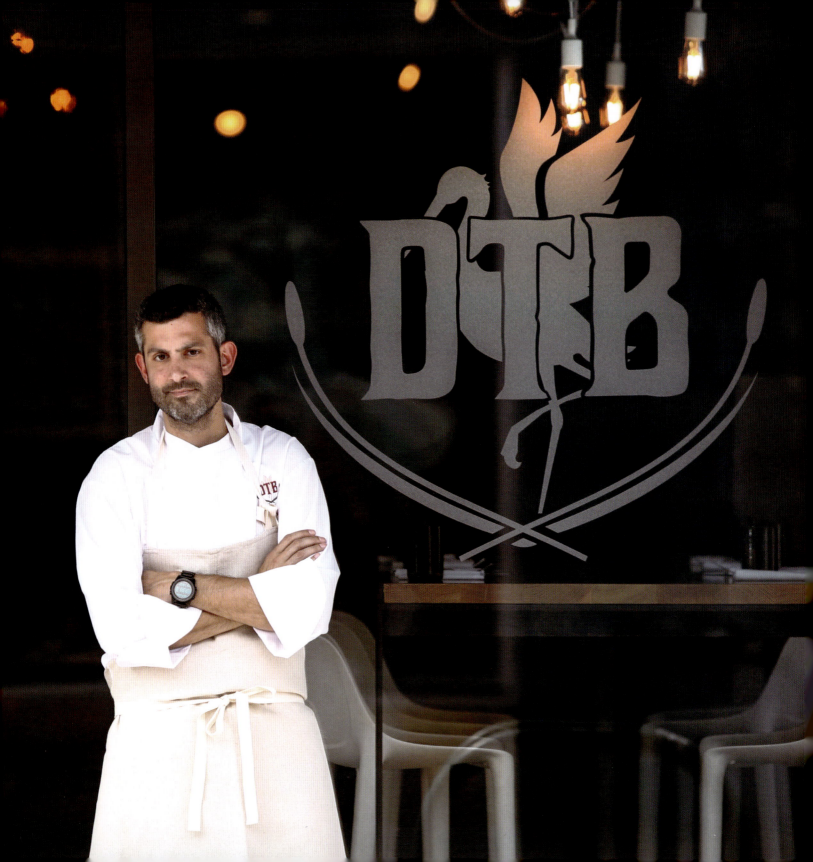

# Chef Carl Schaubhut
## *Eat Fit Chef Ambassador*

Carl and I started working together back in his days as sous chef at Commander's Palace, followed by his time as executive chef for Café Adelaide, a part of the Commander's Family of Restaurants. A brilliant chef and an even more incredible person, Carl embraced Eat Fit from the beginning, welcoming the challenge to integrate nutrition into his restaurants' menus.

Our deeper connection, though, was sparked when Carl was diagnosed with stage 3 esophageal cancer at the age of 31. Along with the full support of Ochsner's oncology team, Carl and his family turned to me for nutritional guidance.

After 9 months of chemo, radiation, and surgery, Carl was back in the kitchen with the drive to really make a difference, nutritionally, on his menus:

> "New Orleans is known for over-the-top abundance. It's part of our DNA: laughing, living, eating, drinking, and I'm grateful to be a part of this, to be a part of people's lives.
>
> As chefs, however, I feel that we have the responsibility to serve food that gives people the opportunity to enjoy a well-planned, artfully crafted dish that's also good for them—and doesn't have to be a special request or burden to the kitchen.
>
> Molly and the Eat Fit team encourage chefs to think about food in a different way than we ever have. It makes me think about food on an even more intense level, beyond just the flavors and ingredients and instead looking at it from a holistic level: how will this make me feel, how it will affect the rest of my day, my energy, my body.
>
> Plus, in the hospitality industry, we're so busy taking care of others that we often don't think about ourselves and our own health. My hope is that along the way, we can change a little bit of this culture as well."

> **"I live my life now to do the right things for myself, my body, my family."**
> —Chef Carl Schaubhut

Carl was the initial inspiration behind the original Eat Fit Cookbook, sparking those very first 'what if' conversations about publishing a collection of restaurant-quality recipes for the home cook.

Re-diagnosed in 2016 with incurable cancer, cooking became a challenge for him—everything became more difficult. His passion for this project continued, though, sending photos of handwritten recipes and prepping and styling the dishes for photo shoots when his energy allowed.

Carl passed away on September 9, 2019—the very day that the proof copies of The Eat Fit Cookbook first arrived from our publisher. He never had the opportunity to hold this book that he gave so much to, but we feel certain that he has seen it, and that he is cheering us on. And we're grateful that his passion and talents continue to fill these pages with love.

(Courtesy Marianna Massey)

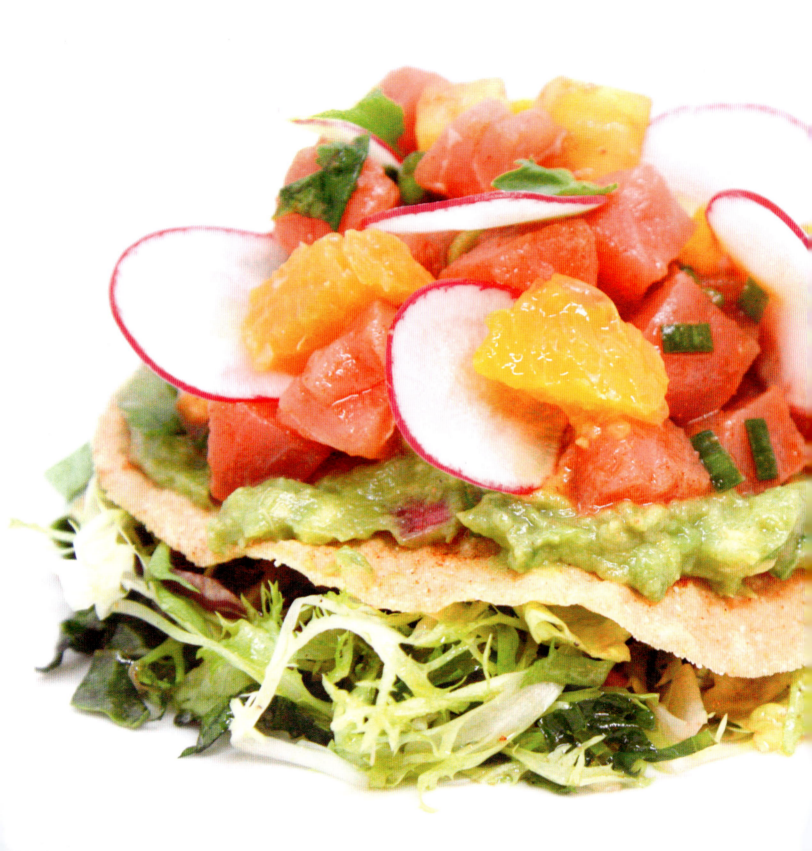

# Yellowfin Tuna Poke Tostada
## Chef Carl Schaubhut

SHARE

**Makes 8 servings**

We are in love with this dish. It is simple, gorgeous, delicate, and worth every step. Don't be intimidated by the long list of ingredients. These layered tostadas are actually super simple to build and much of the prep can be done ahead of time.

- 1½ pounds sushi grade tuna, very cold, diced ½ inch thick
- ½ cup ponzu sauce (recipe follows)
- ½ cup diced fresh pineapple
- 2 oranges, peeled, segmented, and sliced in half
- 1 tablespoon chopped fresh cilantro
- 1 tablespoon chopped fresh basil
- 1 tablespoon chopped green onions
- ½ cup sliced Pickled Red Onions (page 163)
- 1 pinch sea salt
- ¼ teaspoon freshly ground black pepper
- 4 cups mixed greens
- ½ cup rice wine vinaigrette (recipe follows)
- 8 6-inch crispy corn tortilla rounds
- 1 cup guacamole (recipe follows)
- 1 tablespoon black sesame seeds for garnish
- ¼ cup shaved radish for garnish

In a large mixing bowl, combine tuna, ponzu sauce, pineapple, orange segments, cilantro, basil, green onion, pickled red onion, salt, and pepper. Toss gently.

In a second large mixing bowl, toss greens with vinaigrette. Divide greens evenly across 8 plates, forming greens into a tight circle in the center of the plate.

Smear each crispy tortilla with 1-2 tablespoons of guacamole, enough to cover the surface of the tortilla, and place onto plated greens. Spoon the poke mixture on top of guacamole-covered tortillas, sprinkle with sesame seeds and shaved radish, and serve.

PER SERVING: 290 calories, 14 grams fat, 2.5 grams saturated fat, 320 mg sodium, 18 grams carbohydrate (15 grams net carbs), 3 grams fiber, 5 grams sugar (0 added sugar), 23 grams protein

## Chef Tip/

Hearty greens such as Napa cabbage, kale, and frisée work best for this dish.

### PONZU SAUCE

**Makes approximately ½ cup**

2 tablespoons reduced-sodium soy sauce
1 lemon, zested and juiced
1 lime, zested and juiced
1 orange, zested and juiced
½ teaspoon fish sauce

Blend together all ponzu sauce ingredients.

### RICE WINE VINAIGRETTE

**Makes approximately 1½ cups**

½ teaspoon sesame oil
⅓ cup rice vinegar
1 tablespoon reduced sodium soy sauce
½ clove garlic
1 tablespoon minced fresh ginger
½ shallot, peeled
1 tablespoon Dijon mustard
¼ teaspoon fish sauce
¼ teaspoon freshly ground pepper
1 pinch sea salt
1 cup light olive oil

Blend together all ingredients except oil. Slowly add oil to emulsify.

### GUACAMOLE

**Makes approximately 1 cup**

1 avocado, diced
1 lime, zested and juiced
⅛ teaspoon sea salt
2 tablespoons green onion, julienned
¼ red onion, minced
1 clove fresh garlic, minced
2 tablespoons chopped fresh cilantro

Mix all ingredients well. Cover with plastic pressed against guacamole to avoid browning. Set aside until ready to serve.

Brad Schlotterer (Molly's husband) re-creating Chef Carl's Yellowfin Tuna Poke Tostada.

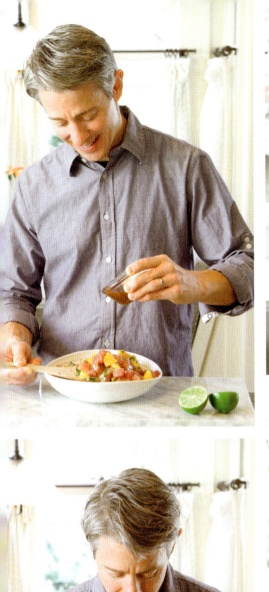
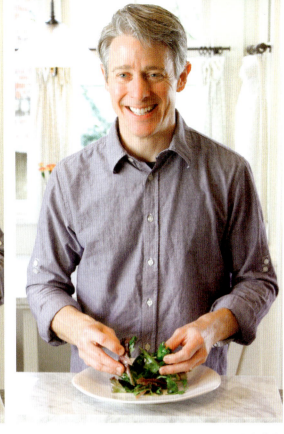
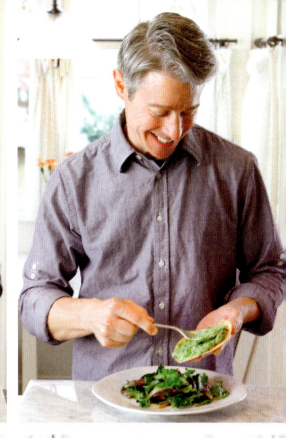
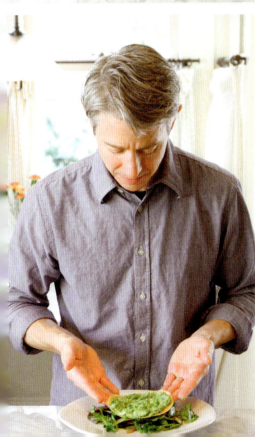
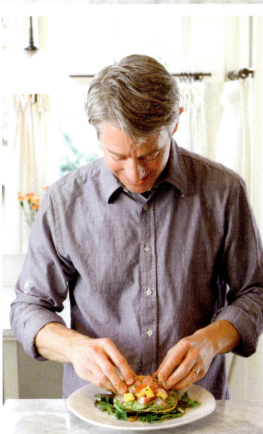
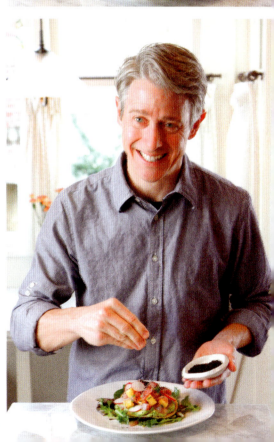

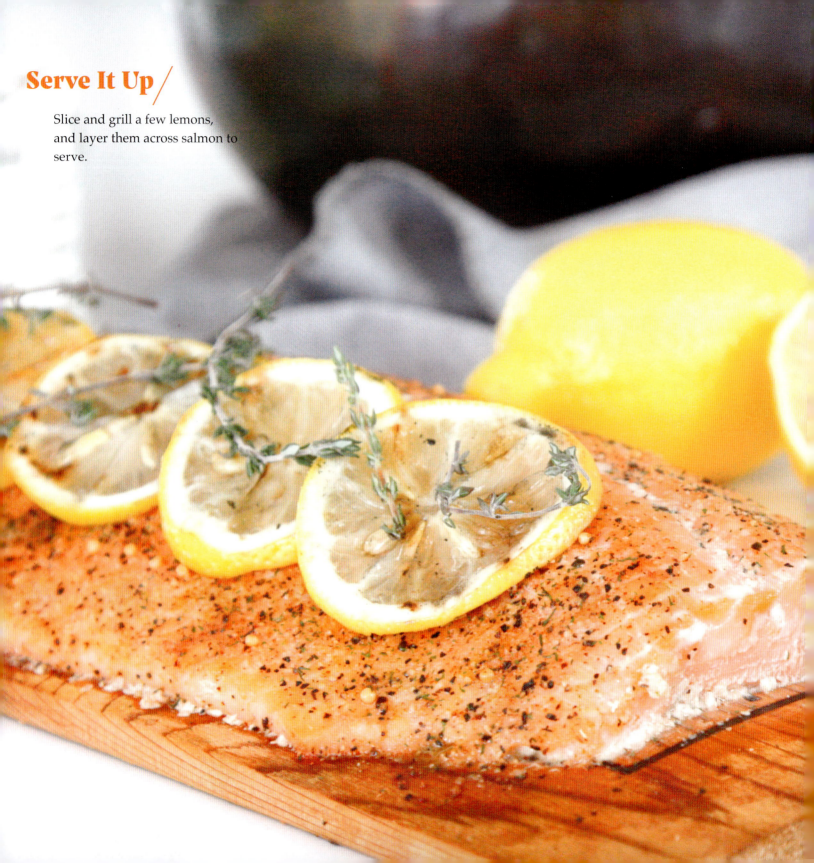

# Serve It Up

Slice and grill a few lemons, and layer them across salmon to serve.

# Cedar Plank Smoked Salmon
*Robért Fresh Market*

**Servings vary**

I love smoked salmon, and Robért Fresh Market's smoked salmon is hands-down the juiciest and most flavorful I've ever had. It's one of my go-to favorites for a girls' night get-together or an impromptu dinner with friends. I love it over whole grain crackers or veggie slices, crumbled over a salad, or added to omelets and frittatas.

**Cedar plank(s)**
**Fresh skinless salmon fillet**
**1 teaspoon light olive oil per 8-12 ounce fillet**
**1 teaspoon Paul Prudhomme's Salmon Magic per 8-12 ounce fillet**

Soak the cedar plank in water for an hour before cooking. Preheat grill or smoker to 250 degrees. If you're using a charcoal grill or smoker, place a small handful of wood chips onto hot coals (for a smokier flavor, soak the chips in water for an hour first).

Rub salmon with olive oil then season with Salmon Magic. Transfer salmon to the soaked cedar plank. Arrange cedar plank carefully on grill so that the coals are on one side of the pit and the salmon plank is on the other.

Cook for 25-30 minutes. Cooking time can range from as little as 20 minutes for a small 4- or 6-ounce fillet to as much as 35 minutes for a full side of salmon. Cook until firm to the touch and internal temperature reaches 145 degrees. Remove from grill or smoker and serve warm, chilled, or at room temperature.

Alternatively, cook in a 350 degree oven for 15-20 minutes. Fish won't have a smoky taste but will pull flavors from the cedar plank.

**PER 4-OUNCE SERVING:** 170 calories, 9 grams fat, 1.5 grams saturated fat, 180 mg sodium, 0 carbohydrate (0 net carbs), 0 fiber, 0 sugar, 22 grams protein
**GF, Low Carb**

## Nutrition Bite

Omega-3s, especially those found in fish oil, are linked to improved mood, brain health, and reduced inflammation. Fish rich in omega-3s can also help to lower blood pressure and triglycerides and protect against certain types of cancer.

## By the Way

Preparing salmon atop a fresh plank of cedar allows us to grill or smoke the fish without it falling apart. It also helps the fish retain its moisture and even pulls flavors from the plank itself.

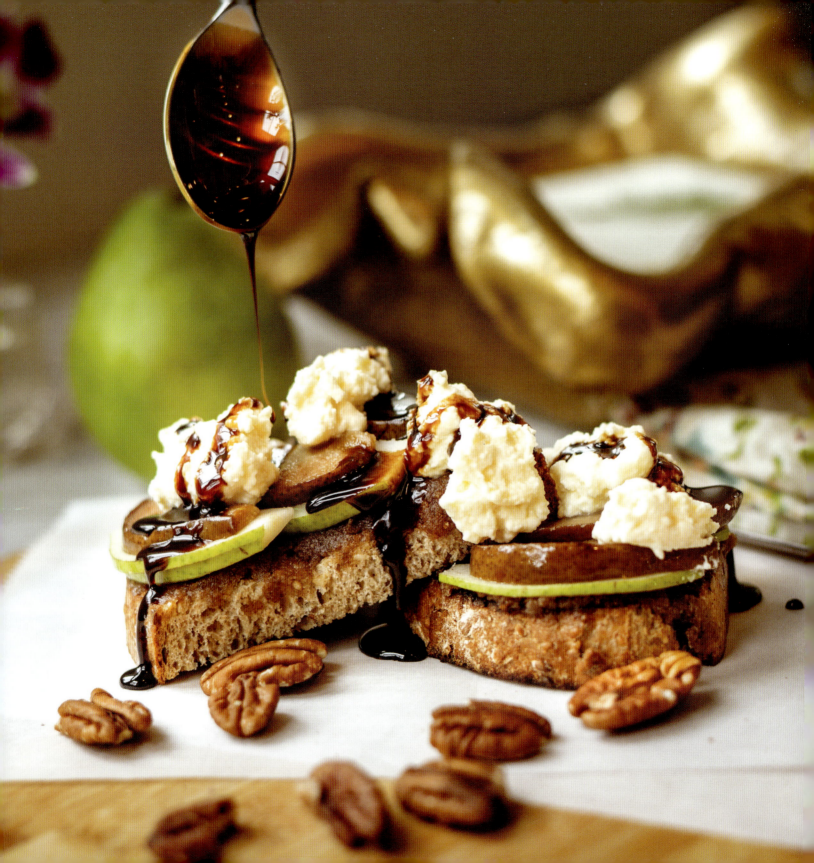

# Pear and Ricotta Tartine with Maple Pecan Butter
## FUEL Café + Market

**Makes 4 servings**

Crunchy, creamy, sweet, savory . . . these all show up and play together so well in this toast built by Chef Ryan Conn of FUEL Café + Market. Serve it for brunch, slice it smaller to serve as an appetizer, or simply keep the prepped ingredients on hand for a quick-yet-indulgent everyday breakfast or snack.

**3 pears**
**4 slices seedy, hearty, artisan-style bread**
**½ cup Maple Pecan Butter (page 187)**
**Whole milk ricotta, the freshest you can find**
**½ cup Balsamic Reduction (recipe follows)**

Preheat oven to 350 degrees. You can prepare the Maple Pecan Butter and Balsamic Reduction in advance, or while pears are baking.

Rinse and cut two of the pears in half lengthwise, from top to bottom. Keep the third pear raw. On a baking sheet lined with parchment paper, place the pears flat side down. Bake for 20 minutes or until just tender to a paring knife (be sure not to over-bake, or skin will wrinkle and pears will be mushy). Remove baking pan from oven and transfer the pears immediately—and carefully—to a cool surface.

Toast the bread in the toaster for a crunch on both sides, or in the oven for a slightly softer side. To assemble the tartine, cut each slice of toast in half, either straight across or as a diagonal. Spread one tablespoon of Maple Pecan Butter onto each piece, pressing gently to give a smooth coating.

With a sharp paring knife, slice the roasted pears into quarter-inch slices lengthwise from top to bottom, working around the core and seeds. Slice the fresh pear so that it is mandolin-thin, even thinner than the poached pears, also lengthwise top to bottom.

In a shingled pattern, arrange the roasted pears and fresh pears—alternating cooked, raw, cooked—over the pecan-buttered toast. Top each with two tablespoon-sized dollops of ricotta. Finally, a graceful drizzle, "as if from the heavens," Chef Ryan says, of the Balsamic Reduction. Serve immediately.

**PER 4-OUNCE SERVING:** 380 calories, 23 grams fat, 4.5 grams saturated fat, 240 mg sodium, 37 grams carbohydrate (27 grams net carbs), 10 grams fiber, 19 grams sugar (0 added sugar), 10 grams protein

VEGETARIAN

### BALSAMIC REDUCTION
**1 cup balsamic vinegar**

In a small saucepan on low heat, simmer balsamic vinegar, stirring occasionally, for about 20 minutes until it thickens enough to coat the back of a spoon, a little thicker than maple syrup. The vinegar will cook down to about one-third or one-half of the volume.

## How We Slice It

Choice of bread is up to you—we prefer a seedy whole grain or a quality gluten free bread (like Base Culture), depending on preference and need.

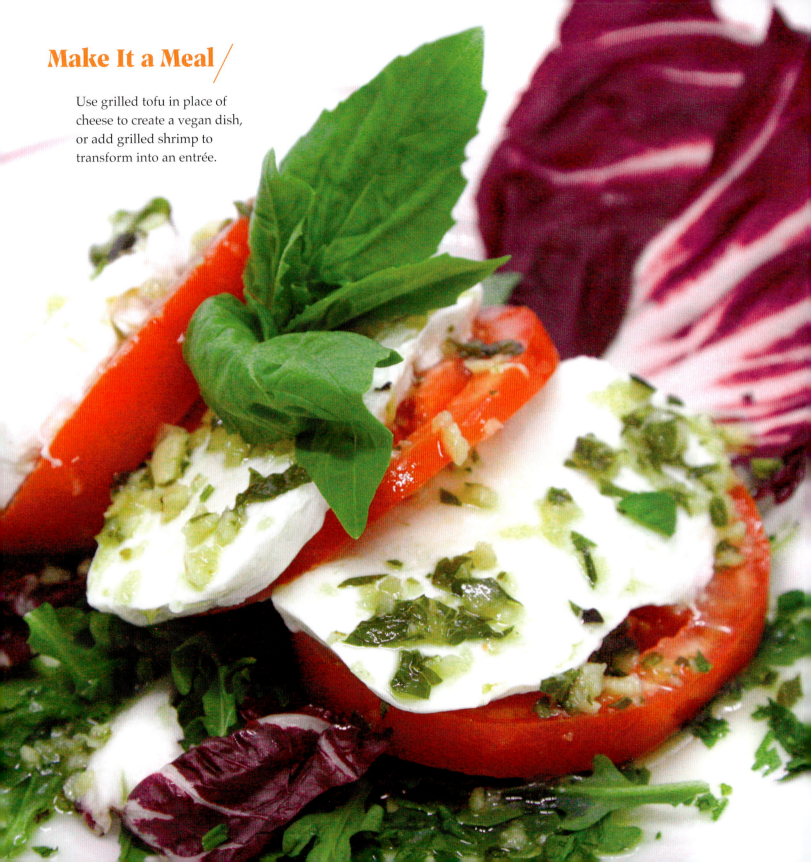

# Make It a Meal /

Use grilled tofu in place of cheese to create a vegan dish, or add grilled shrimp to transform into an entrée.

# Insalate Caprese
## Andrea's Restaurant

**Makes 8 servings**

Beautifully presented and surprisingly simple, this salad is a timeless classic.

2 cups mixed baby greens
1 tablespoon extra virgin olive oil
1 dash sea salt
4 Creole tomatoes, cut into ½-inch slices
½ pound fresh mozzarella, sliced into 16 thin slices
½ cup Fresh Basil Vinaigrette (page 172)
4 purple cabbage leaves, torn in half, for garnish
8 leaves fresh basil for garnish

Lightly coat greens with olive oil and salt, then divide evenly over 8 salad plates. Top each plate with alternating slices of tomato and mozzarella (2 slices of each) and finish with a drizzle (about 1 tablespoon) of dressing. Garnish with purple cabbage leaves and fresh basil.

**PER SERVING:** 230 calories, 20 grams fat, 5 grams saturated fat, 320 mg sodium, 6 grams carbohydrate (5 grams net carbs), 1 gram fiber, 3 grams sugar (0 added sugar), 8 grams protein
GF, LOW CARB, VEGETARIAN

## Serve It Up

Creamy burrata or goat cheese can take the place of fresh mozzarella, and multi-hued heirloom tomatoes can be layered in for color.

## Chef Tip

The fresh mozzarella slices should be very thin, because we want multiple layers without getting too cheesy (translation: keeping animal fats in check). To achieve nice flat slices, be sure your knife is super sharp and the mozzarella ball has been chilled.

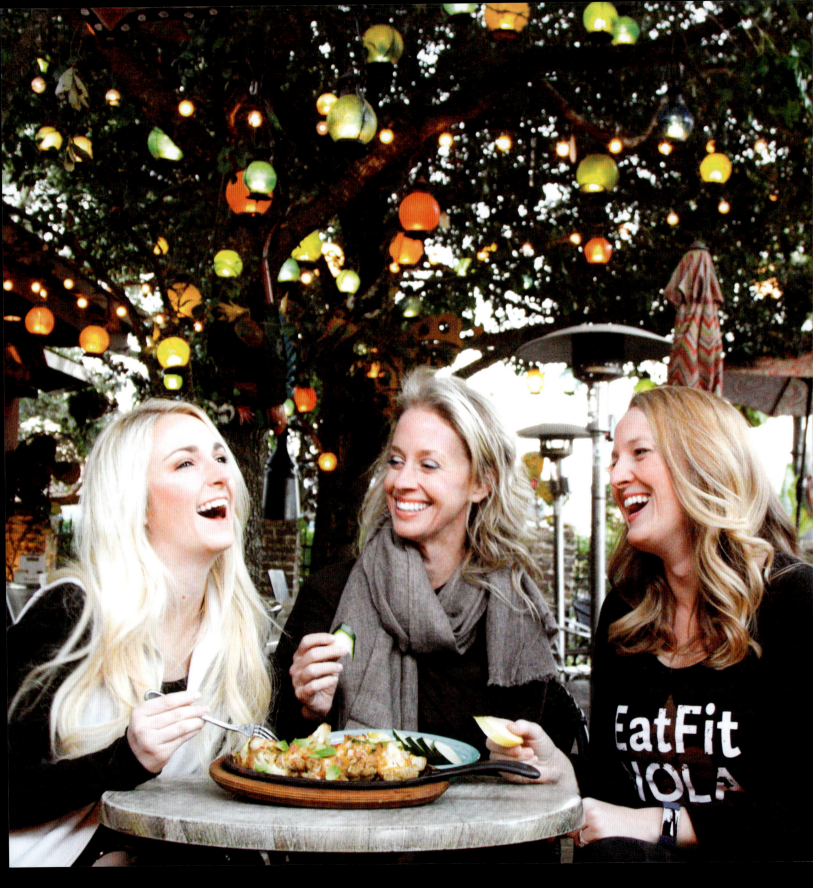

# Cauliflower Nachos
## The Velvet Cactus

**Makes 4 servings**

Low-carb nachos are now a reality in our life! When you are craving this classic Mexican appetizer but don't want the carbs, try this dish on for size. The Velvet Cactus turns up the heat with this healthy take on a spicy nacho plate.

### For the Pico de Gallo
- 1 medium red tomato, seeded and diced
- 1 yellow onion, diced
- 1 fresh jalapeño, seeded and diced
- ¼ cup chopped fresh cilantro
- 2 tablespoons lime juice
- 1 teaspoon minced fresh garlic
- Pinch of sea salt
- ½ teaspoon freshly ground black pepper

### For the Nachos
- 6 cups cauliflower florets
- 2 tablespoons extra virgin olive oil
- ½ teaspoon garlic powder
- ½ teaspoon chili powder
- ½ teaspoon cumin
- ¼ teaspoon sea salt
- ½ cup chopped red bell pepper
- ½ cup sliced fresh jalapeños
- ⅓ cup shredded cheddar cheese
- ½ avocado, sliced

**Prepare the Pico de Gallo:** Combine all pico de gallo ingredients in a large mixing bowl. Set aside. Pico de gallo can be refrigerated for up to 4 days.

**Assemble the Nachos:** Place cauliflower in a pot and fill with water to cover half of the cauliflower. Steam, covered, for 7-10 minutes or until soft. Place cauliflower in an ice bath. Remove and pat gently to dry.

Add oil to a grill pan and heat to medium heat. Sprinkle steamed cauliflower with garlic powder, chili powder, cumin, and sea salt. Grill for about 5 minutes, until browned.

In a mixing bowl, combine the browned cauliflower, pico de gallo, and peppers. Transfer the mixture to a cast-iron skillet or other oven-safe serving dish. Top with shredded cheese and broil until browned. Garnish with avocado slices and serve.

**PER SERVING:** 200 calories, 14 grams fat, 3.5 grams saturated fat, 230 mg sodium, 18 grams carbohydrate (11 grams net carbs), 7 grams fiber, 7 grams sugar (0 added sugar), 7 grams protein
GF, Vegetarian

From left: Eat Fit NOLA's Lauren Berry, Molly, and Rebecca Miller.

### Serve It Up
Dial up your presentation by serving in a cast-iron skillet.

### Love It Later
In the unlikely event of leftovers, these "nachos" are delish stir-fried with shrimp or chicken.

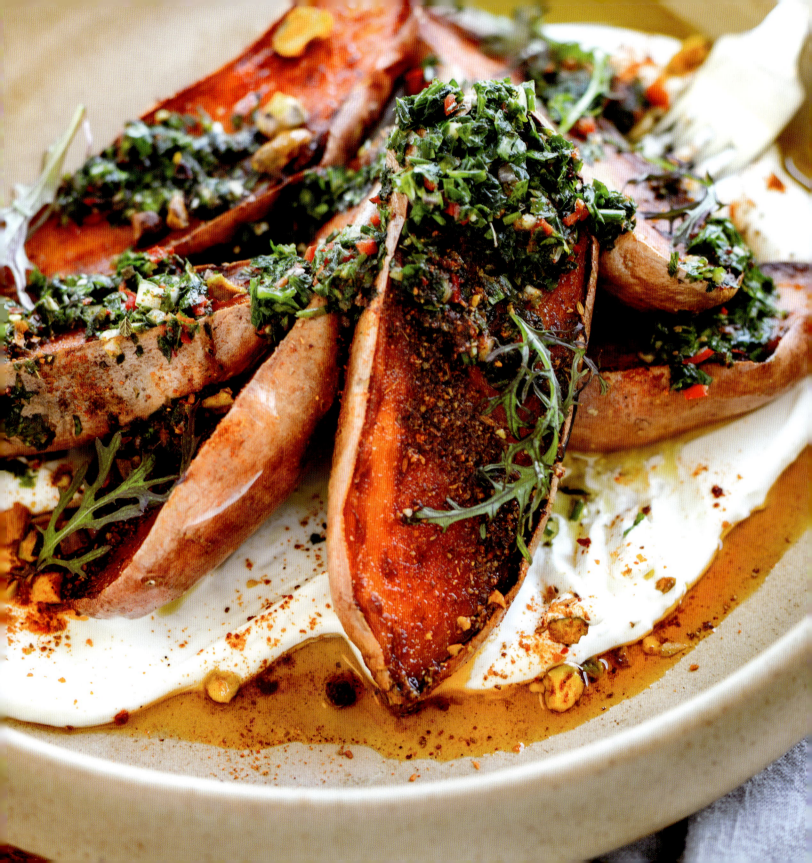

# Caramelized Sweet Potato with Labneh and Chimichurri
## *Parish Restaurant*

**Makes 4-6 servings**

Herbaceous and lovely with satisfyingly crispy edges and buttery soft goodness inside, Chef Corey Bahr takes the savory route with these darling little sweets.

**6 small sweet potatoes, like fingerlings**
**1 tablespoon grapeseed or extra virgin olive oil**
**Pinch of sea salt**
**1/2 cup Labneh (page 174)**
**2 tablespoons Chimichurri (page 184)**

Preheat oven to 400 degrees. Wash sweet potatoes and cut in half lengthwise. Brush with oil and sprinkle with salt. On a baking sheet lined with parchment paper, place cut side down and roast for 25-35 minutes, until caramelized and tender.

Once potatoes are cooled, spoon the Labneh onto a serving platter and spread across to create a thin layer. Pile sweet potatoes on top; finish with a drizzle of Chimichurri and serve.

**PER SERVING:** 190 calories, 7 grams fat, 1.5 grams saturated fat, 220 mg sodium, 29 grams carbohydrate (25 grams net carbs), 4 grams fiber, 6 grams sugar (0 added sugar), 4 grams protein
**GF**

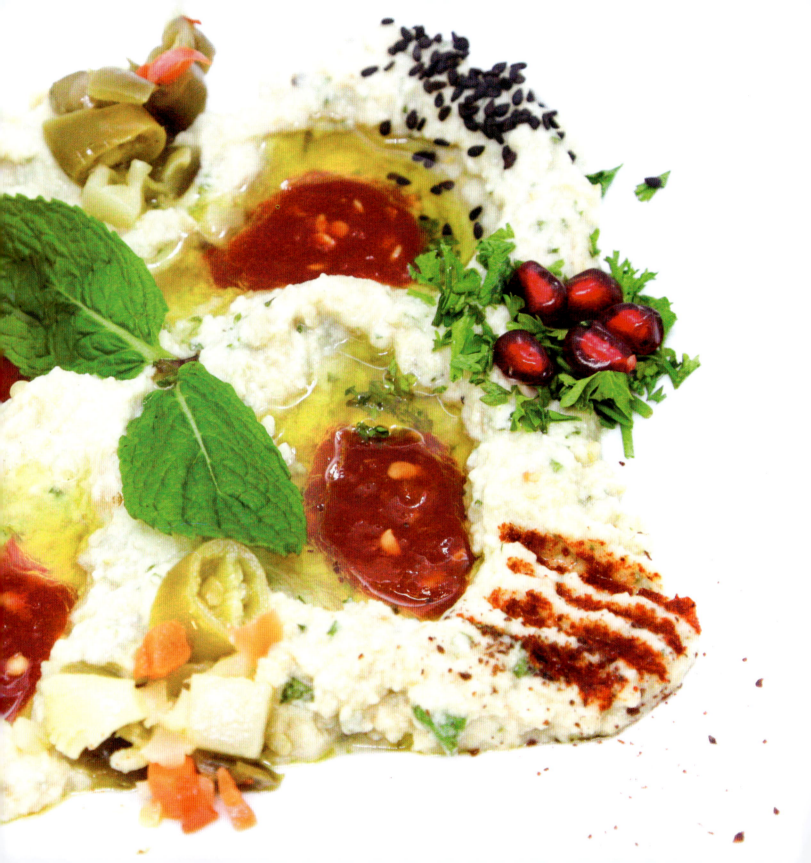

# Baba Ganoush
## Cleo's Mediterranean Cuisine & Grocery

**Makes 8 servings**

Greek yogurt is the secret ingredient in Cleo's creamy Baba Ganoush, but it can easily be omitted to create a vegan alternative. Pair it with lean protein for dipping or serve as an appetizer or side dish with raw veggies. Our favorite dipping vehicles include celery and thick-sliced yellow and red peppers.

- 1 large eggplant
- 1 tablespoon extra virgin olive oil
- ¼ cup 2% plain Greek yogurt
- ¼ cup tahini
- 2 cloves garlic, minced
- ¼ cup lemon juice
- ¼ cup chopped fresh parsley
- ½ teaspoon sea salt

**For the Garnish**
- 1 tablespoon chili paste
- 2 tablespoons extra virgin olive oil
- ¼ teaspoon black sesame seeds
- 1 small fresh jalapeño, sliced
- 1 tablespoon chopped fresh parsley
- 1 teaspoon fresh pomegranate seeds (substitute diced red pepper or fresh raspberries)
- 1 sprig fresh mint

Preheat oven to 375 degrees and heat grill to medium-hot. Prick eggplant with a fork and place onto grill rack 4-5 inches from the fire. (Don't feel like going outside to grill? Use your broiler instead.) Grill, turning frequently, until the skin blackens, blisters, and begins to soften, approximately 10-15 minutes.

Transfer eggplant to a baking sheet, cover with foil, and bake until very soft, about 20 minutes. Remove from oven, let cool slightly, then remove the skin.

Place the eggplant flesh into a food processor and blend until a paste forms. Add olive oil, yogurt, tahini, garlic, lemon juice, parsley, and salt and mix well.

Transfer the mixture to a serving bowl or plate. Smooth the mixture with the back of a spoon and press lightly to form 4 shallow wells. Fill wells with half a tablespoon each of chili paste and olive oil. Garnish with small clusters of black sesame seeds, jalapeño slices, and chopped parsley topped with pomegranate seeds. Top with fresh mint and serve.

**PER SERVING:** 120 calories, 10 grams fat, 1.5 grams saturated fat, 170 mg sodium, 8 grams carbohydrate (5 grams net carbs), 3 grams fiber, 3 grams sugar (<1 gram added sugar), 3 grams protein
GF, Low Carb, Vegetarian

## Nutrition Bite

Use peeled, puréed eggplant to add thickness and richness to just about any creamy dip.

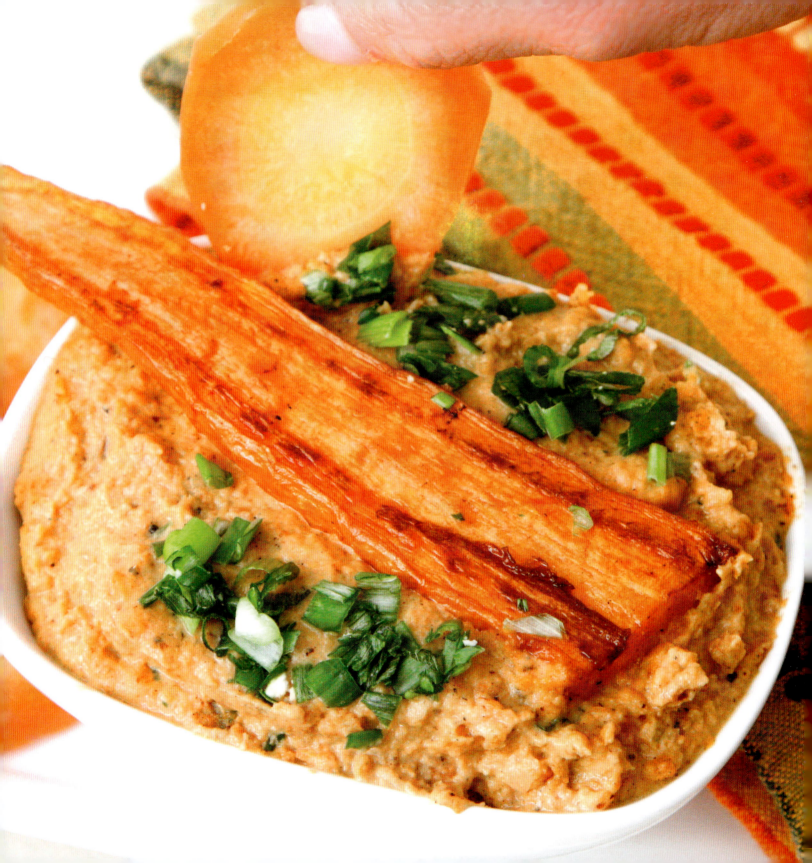

# Carrot Hummus
## *Mestizo Louisiana Mexican Cuisine*

**Makes 6 servings**

We love non-traditional spins on tried-and-true dishes. Carrot hummus is a brightly colored alternative that slashes the carby calories and boosts the nutritional benefits of regular hummus.

1 large carrot, peeled and thinly sliced
1 clove garlic, chopped
¼ medium onion, chopped
1 Roma tomato, quartered and seeded
¼ Serrano pepper, sliced
2 tablespoons extra virgin olive oil, divided
1 cup cooked garbanzo beans, drained
1 tablespoon tahini
½ teaspoon sea salt

Preheat oven to 400 degrees. On a large baking sheet, place carrot, garlic, onion, tomato, and Serrano pepper and drizzle with 1 tablespoon olive oil. Roast for 15 minutes. Remove from oven, turn vegetables, then cover with foil and return to oven for an additional 10-15 minutes, until carrots are soft. Remove from oven and cool.

Place garbanzo beans, tahini, salt, and remaining olive oil into a blender and blend until smooth. Slowly add roasted vegetables and blend slowly until smooth. Serve immediately or cover and refrigerate for later.

**PER SERVING (2 TABLESPOONS):** 110 calories, 7 grams fat, 1 gram saturated fat, 190 mg sodium, 11 grams carbohydrate (8 grams net carbs), 3 grams fiber, 3 grams sugar (0 added sugar), 3 grams protein
GF, Low Carb, Vegan

## Serve It Up /

Delicious with unique dippers like jicama and red peppers, as a spread for sandwiches and wraps, or atop lean proteins such as chicken and pork.

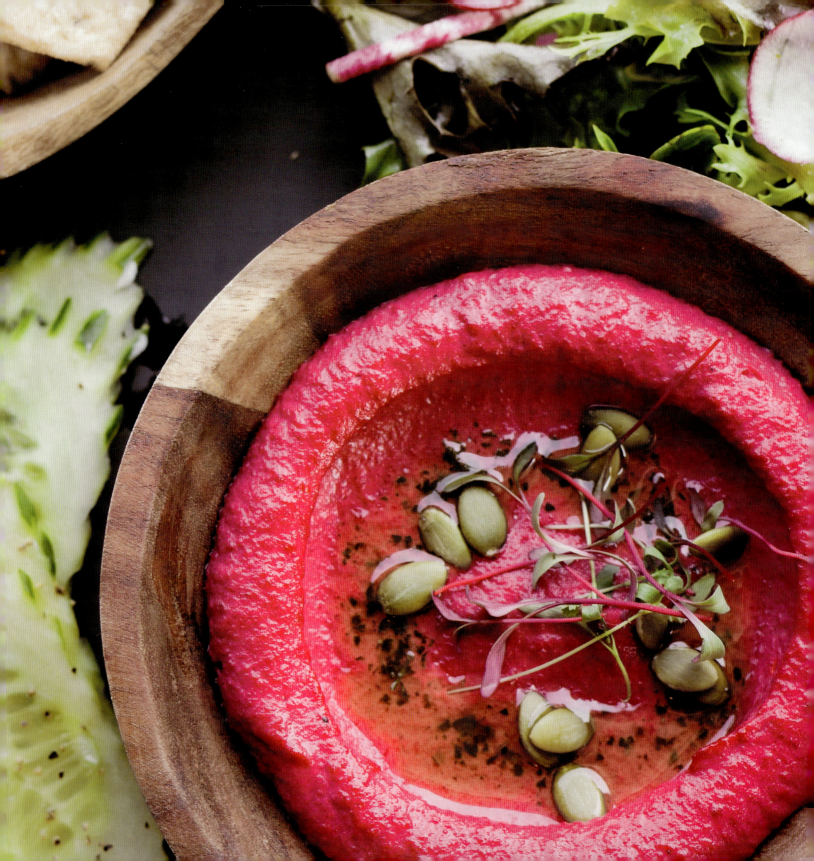

# Beet Hummus
## Cured. On Columbia

**Makes 16 servings**

Chef Amanda, co-owner of Cured. On Columbia, never ate beets as a kid. You know how it goes—her mom didn't like beets, so she thought she didn't like them. As an adult though, she grew to love beets, and this dish was born, giving us the perfect balance of sweet and spicy and just a bit of earthiness. As for her mom? This beet hummus just may have converted her.

4 large beets
Olive oil
⅔ cup tahini paste
2 lemons, zested and juiced
8 cloves of Confit Garlic (recipe follows)
1 teaspoon cane vinegar
1 tablespoon honey
1 teaspoon Cured. House Seasoning (recipe follows)
1 teaspoon red pepper flakes
⅓ cup Confit Garlic Oil (recipe follows)
1 pinch of salt

Preheat oven to 350 degrees. Wash whole beets and place in roasting pan. Cover generously with olive oil and roast for 25-30 minutes or until soft enough to pierce with a fork. Let cool, then peel and chop.

Combine beets, tahini, lemon juice, lemon zest, Confit Garlic, cane vinegar, honey, Cured. House Seasoning, and red pepper flakes in a food processor and start to blend.

While blending, slowly drizzle in the Confit Garlic Oil and continue to blend until smooth. Add a tablespoon of hot water if needed to achieve desired consistency.

Taste and adjust seasoning as needed; add more olive oil, lemon juice, or salt if desired.

Serve in a bowl with your favorite toppings (Chef Amanda loves pepitas, microgreens, goat cheese, and honey drizzle) and the remaining Confit Garlic Oil.

**PER SERVING:** 120 calories, 10 grams fat, 1.5 grams saturated fat, 50 mg sodium, 6 grams carbohydrate (5 grams net carbs), 1 gram fiber, 3 grams sugar (1 gram added sugar), 2 grams protein

GF, Low Carb, Vegetarian, Low Sodium

## CONFIT GARLIC + GARLIC OIL

8 garlic cloves
½ cup olive oil

In a small, shallow, oven safe dish, add garlic cloves and cover with olive oil. Roast at 350 for 15 minutes or until garlic is browned and super fragrant. Do not overcook. Save any remaining Confit Garlic Oil in an airtight container.

## CURED. HOUSE SEASONING BLEND

1 teaspoon sea salt
1 teaspoon garlic powder
1 teaspoon onion powder
1 teaspoon black pepper
½ teaspoon cayenne

Combine all seasonings in a bowl. If pressed for time, can use low-sodium Cajun seasoning blend.

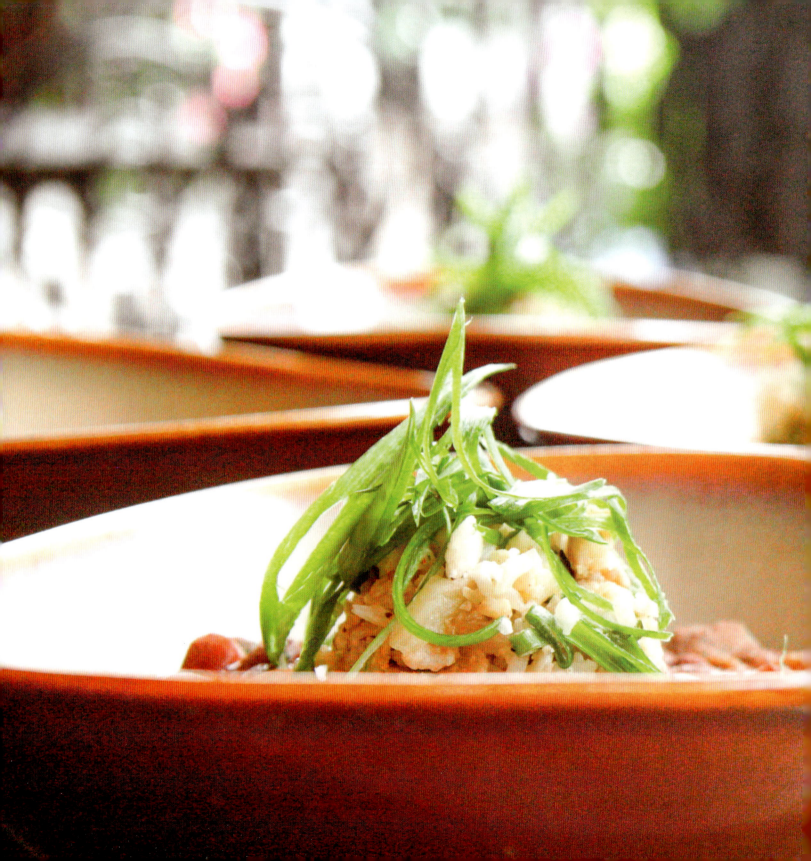

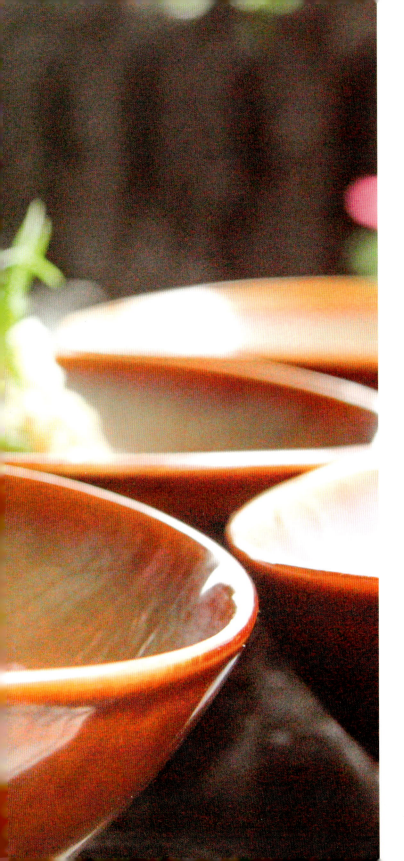

# 2
# BOWLS
## Bisques, Soups + Spoonables

Whether we love them for cultural, seasonal, or sentimental reasons, comfort foods warm us from within. Unfortunately, they're not always (okay, almost never) nutritious, but our recipes are the exception. These nourishing bisques, soups, and spoonables are colorful, creative, and carefully crafted by Eat Fit chefs to maintain the integrity and taste of both traditional and not-so-traditional comfort foods.

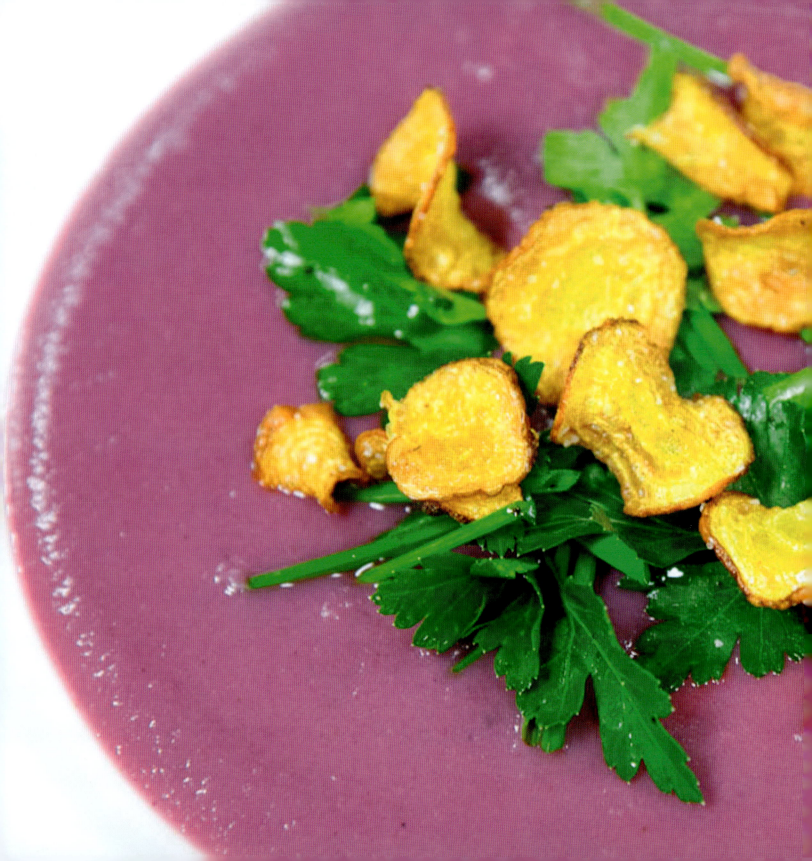

# Sweet Potato Carnival Soup
## Commander's Palace

**Makes 12 servings**

While New Orleans is famously regarded for its exquisite cuisine, the city is also known worldwide for its endearingly boisterous Carnival season. Chef Meg Bickford of Commander's Palace created this hearty, colorful vegan soup that merges the classic flavors of New Orleans cuisine with the colors of Mardi Gras.

- 3 pounds purple sweet potatoes
- 2 tablespoons light olive oil
- 1 small onion, chopped
- 1 small shallot, chopped
- 2 cloves garlic, chopped
- 1 teaspoon paprika
- ½ teaspoon cayenne pepper
- ½ teaspoon cinnamon
- 5 sprigs thyme
- ¼ bunch parsley
- 2 bay leaves
- ¾ teaspoon salt
- 2 quarts unsalted vegetable stock
- ¾ cup lemon juice
- 1 teaspoon Steen's cane vinegar
- Beet Medallions for garnish (page 164)

Preheat oven to 425 degrees. Pierce each purple sweet potato with a fork 2-3 times and spread onto baking sheet (no need to wrap with foil). Bake for 45 minutes to 1 hour (a little longer if they're super large). Turn off oven and allow sweet potatoes to sit in hot oven for at least 30 minutes. Remove sweet potatoes from oven, peel the skin, cut into large cubes, and set aside.

In a large pot over medium heat, add oil and sauté onion, shallot, and garlic until translucent. Add purple sweet potatoes, paprika, cayenne, cinnamon, thyme, parsley, bay leaves, and salt and sauté until fragrant. Add vegetable stock and bring to a simmer. Simmer for 10 minutes, stirring occasionally. Remove bay leaves and puree soup until smooth using an immersion blender. Add lemon juice and vinegar, garnish with Beet Medallions, and serve.

**PER SERVING:** 190 calories, 2.5 grams fat, 0 saturated fat, 290 mg sodium, 37 grams carbohydrate (32 grams net carbs), 5 grams fiber, 9 grams sugar (0 added sugar), 3 grams protein

GF, Vegan

## Tip

Don't have an immersion blender? A food processor will work just fine.

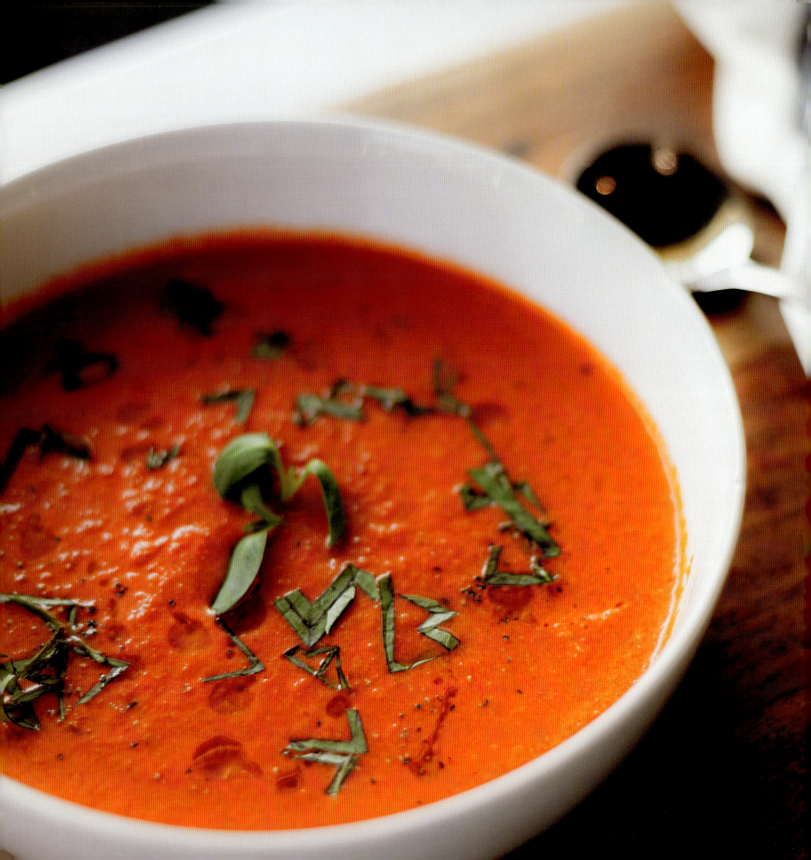

# Smoked Tomato Basil Soup
## Cured. On Columbia

**Makes 6-8 servings**

Comfort food that's elevated and nourishing. We love this soup paired with a good-for-you savory grilled cheese, or a crispy summertime salad. It's also an excellent make-ahead "veggie" for any weeknight dinner.

Wood chips
2 tomatoes, roughly chopped
3 tablespoons extra virgin olive oil, divided
2 teaspoons Cured. House Seasoning Blend, divided (page 45)
¼ onion, chopped
8 ounces Rotel tomatoes
1 can (14 ounces) crushed tomatoes
2 garlic cloves, peeled
2 ounces Parmigiano Reggiano, cut into small chunks
½ cup heavy whipping cream
¼ cup fresh basil leaves, loose, not packed, plus more for garnish
¼ teaspoon red pepper flakes
¼ teaspoon sea salt

If smoking in an oven, preheat oven to 275 degrees. If using oven, soak wood chips in water for several hours, then drain. Place the chips in the bottom of an aluminum roasting pan in a single layer. Pour just enough of the soaking liquid to cover the chips. In a metal pan, toss chopped tomatoes with 1 tablespoon of olive oil and 1 teaspoon of House Seasoning Blend. Place tomatoes on a roasting rack on top of the wood chips. Smoke for 3 hours in oven, or in a smoker.

To prepare the soup, sauté onions in 2 tablespoons of olive oil in a large stock pot over medium-high heat, until translucent. Stir in smoked tomatoes, Rotel tomatoes, crushed tomatoes, and garlic. Bring to a light boil, stirring occasionally and allow to simmer for 30 minutes.

Add Parmigiano Reggiano. Stir until melted throughout, then add heavy whipping cream, fresh basil, red pepper flakes, and 1 teaspoon of House Seasoning Blend and sea salt. Blend with immersion blender until desired texture. Garnish with remaining fresh basil.

**PER SERVING:** 180 calories, 15 grams fat, 6 grams saturated fat, 430 mg sodium, 9 grams carbohydrate (7 grams net carbs), 2 gram fiber, 5 grams sugar, 6 grams protein
GF, Low Carb

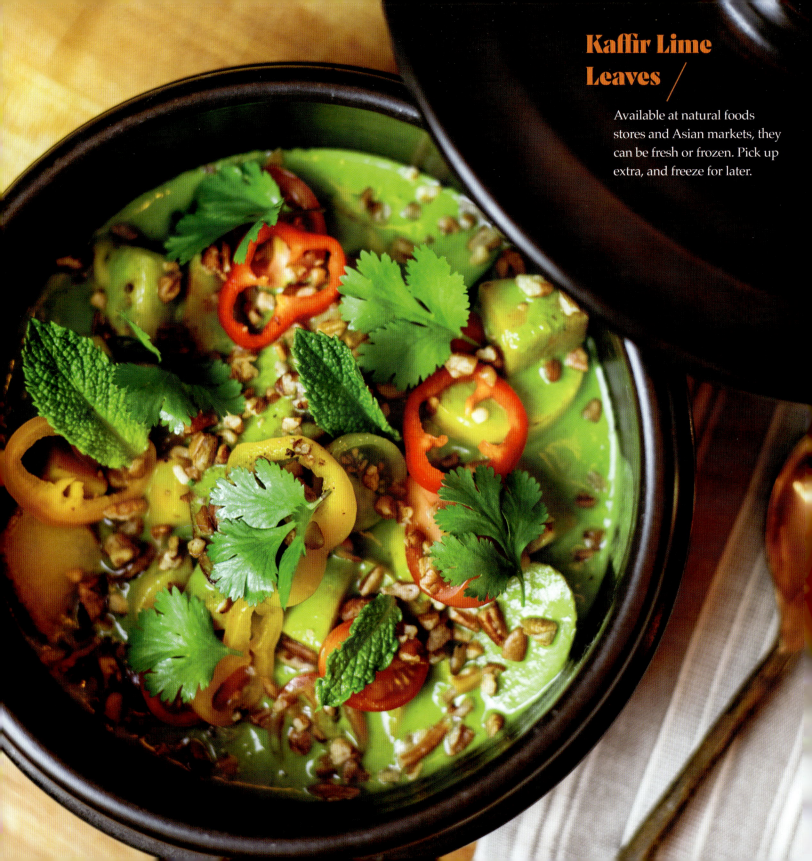

## Kaffir Lime Leaves

Available at natural foods stores and Asian markets, they can be fresh or frozen. Pick up extra, and freeze for later.

# Thai Green Curry
## Miss River

**Makes 4 servings**

Aromatic and bright with a delicate heat on the finish, this recipe is simply a guide to get you started. Don't limit yourself to the ingredients on the page below—this dish can be made with limitless combinations of fresh, seasonal vegetables. Some of our other favorites include asparagus, mushrooms, cauliflower, and fresh wilted spinach. Add shrimp or chicken, or keep it vegan with cubes of firm tofu.

1 teaspoon olive oil
3 tablespoons minced shallot
1 tablespoon minced garlic
9 Tinkerbell mini red bell peppers, sliced into thin rings (or any variety of small red or yellow bell pepper)
2 small Thai or Japanese eggplants, thinly sliced into half-moons
1 zucchini squash, cut into bite-sized pieces
6 cups Green Curry Base (recipe follows)
20 cherry tomatoes, halved
8 sprigs fresh cilantro
12 mint leaves (torn to medium pieces)
4 tablespoons toasted pecan pieces
2 fresh limes, halved lengthwise

In a large pot over medium heat, add oil, shallots, garlic, and peppers and cook for 2 minutes. Add eggplant and zucchini squash and cook for another 3 minutes. Add Green Curry Base and bring to a simmer. Add cherry tomatoes and remove from heat. Distribute evenly into 4 bowls. Serve topped with fresh herbs, pecans, and lime.

**PER SERVING:** 480 calories, 37 grams fat, 20 grams saturated fat, 640 mg sodium, 34 grams carbohydrate (25 grams net carbs), 9 grams fiber, 13 grams sugar (0 added sugar), 8 grams protein
**GF, VEGAN**

### GREEN CURRY BASE

4 tablespoons olive oil
2 tablespoons unsalted green curry paste
2 tablespoons minced lemongrass
4½ tablespoons minced ginger
2 tablespoons minced garlic clove
5 teaspoons jalapeño pepper, seeded and minced
1½ teaspoons lemon zest
½ teaspoon ground star anise
½ teaspoon ground allspice
4 cups low sodium vegetable stock
10 kaffir lime leaves
2 bay leaves
2½ cups coconut milk
1½ teaspoons salt
2½ tablespoons cornstarch
2½ tablespoons water
2 bunches parsley
1 cup chopped green onion

Over low heat in a large heavy bottom pot, add oil and green curry paste and sweat lemongrass, ginger, garlic, and jalapeño with the lemon zest, star anise, and allspice until soft. Add vegetable stock, lime leaves, bay leaves, coconut milk, and salt and bring to a simmer. Cook on low for 1 hour. Remove lime leaves and bay leaves.

Make a slurry with the cornstarch and water and add to the base, stirring until well-incorporated. Remove from heat and allow to cool. Blend parsley and green onions into the base with an immersion blender until fully incorporated. Strain through a fine mesh strainer, making sure to press all solids until dry.

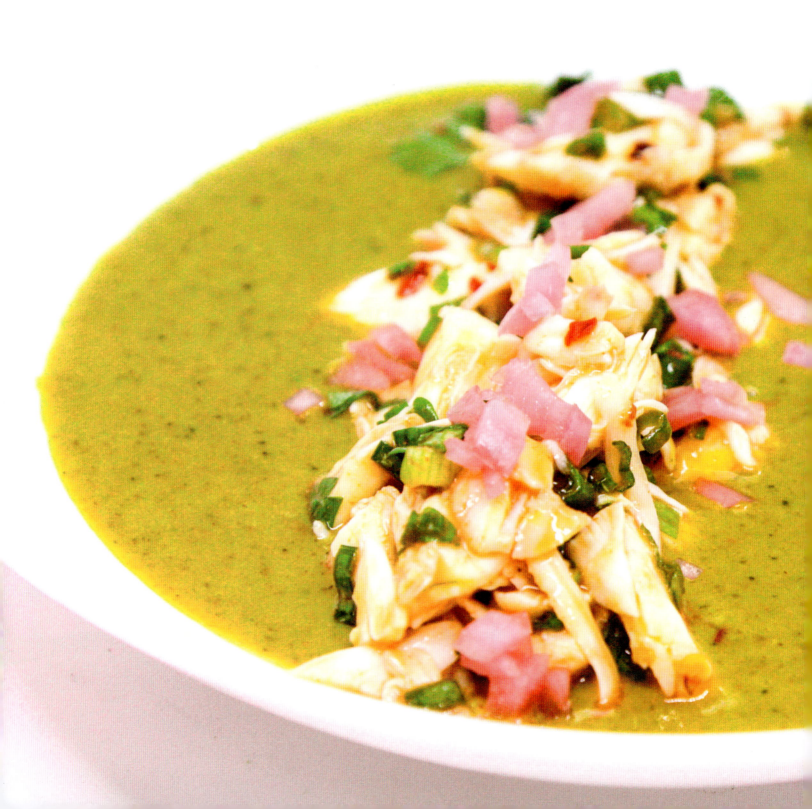

# Curried Carrot + Coconut Soup with Jumbo Lump Crab + Lime

*Chef Carl Schaubhut*

**Makes 8 servings**

The many sophisticated flavors of curry and coconut paired with zesty lemongrass are a testament to Chef Carl's culinary talent.

- 1 tablespoon light olive oil
- 1 yellow onion, chopped
- 3 celery ribs, chopped
- 2 medium yellow bell peppers, chopped
- ¼ cup fresh ginger, peeled and sliced
- 2 stalks lemongrass, smashed
- 4 garlic cloves, smashed
- ¼ teaspoon sea salt
- 1 teaspoon ground black pepper
- 1 tablespoon curry powder
- 1 teaspoon low-sodium Creole seasoning
- 1 teaspoon dried basil
- ¼ cup rice wine
- 8 cups unsalted vegetable stock
- 2½ cups chopped carrots
- 1 cup coconut cream
- 1 cup canned unsweetened coconut milk
- 3 tablespoons hot sauce
- 2 tablespoons Lea & Perrins Worcestershire sauce
- 1 lime, juiced and zested
- 1 batch Jumbo Lump Crab + Lime Topping (recipe follows)

In a large pot over medium heat, add oil and sauté onion, celery, yellow pepper, ginger, lemongrass, and garlic. Mix in salt and pepper. Cook for 15 minutes, stirring frequently until onion is translucent. Add curry powder, Creole seasoning, and basil.

Deglaze the pot with rice wine. Add stock and carrots and bring to a boil. Reduce to a simmer and cook for 20 minutes, until carrots are tender. Remove lemongrass and discard. Puree mixture in small batches with an immersion blender or in a food processor and return to pot. Add coconut cream and milk, hot sauce, Worcestershire, and lime. Stir to combine.

Serve soup hot or chilled, topped with ¼ cup Jumbo Lump Crab + Lime Topping.

**PER SERVING:** 270 calories, 19 grams fat, 15 grams saturated fat, 540 mg sodium, 15 grams carbohydrate (12 grams net carbs), 3 grams fiber, 4 grams sugar (<1 gram added sugar), 15 grams protein

## Serve It Up

The crabmeat topping is also delicious atop bib lettuce or toasted whole grain crostini.

### JUMBO LUMP CRAB + LIME TOPPING

**Makes 8 servings**

- 1 pound jumbo lump crabmeat
- 2 tablespoons reduced sodium soy sauce
- 1 teaspoon sriracha
- ¼ cup Steen's cane vinegar
- ¼ teaspoon fish sauce
- 1 lime, zested
- 2 tablespoons chopped cilantro
- 1 bunch green onions, thinly sliced

Place all ingredients in a large bowl and gently mix until well combined. Chill before serving.

## By the Way /

Creole seasoning is an all-in-one type of seasoning created and made popular by Chef Paul Prudhomme in the Commander's Palace kitchen. Chef Paul was known for cooking with multiple blends of dried herbs, spices, dehydrated vegetable powders, and dried chili powders.

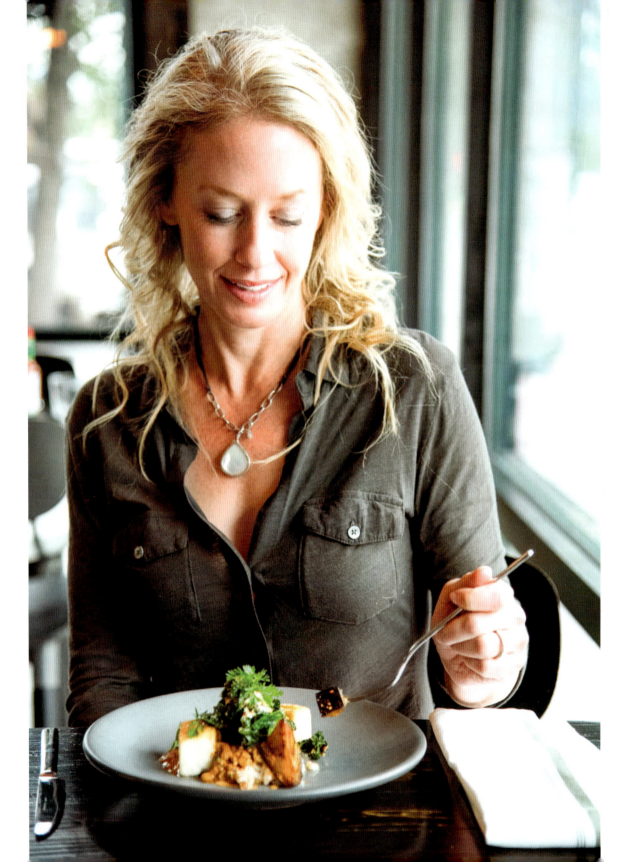

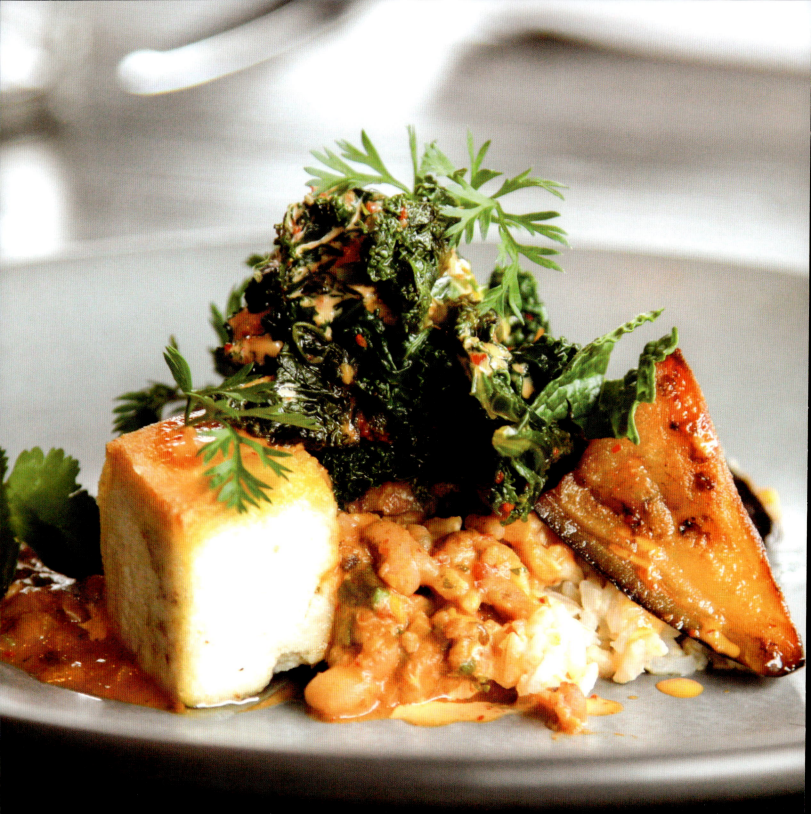

# Tofu + Eggplant in Field Pea Curry
*MoPho*

**Makes 6 servings**

Chef Michael Gulotta's attention to detail in every element of this plant-based dish allows the flavors and textures to shine through deliciously. Eggplant lends a rich, meaty quality without adding a ton of calories and carbs.

**For the Roasted Garlic Vinaigrette**
- 1½ cups light olive oil, divided
- ½ head garlic, peeled
- 1 small shallot, minced
- 1-inch ginger root, peeled and grated
- ½ cup seasoned rice wine vinegar
- ½ tablespoon Sambal chili paste
- ½ tablespoon peanut butter
- ½ tablespoon sesame oil

**For the Eggplant + Tofu Salad**
- ¼ cup light olive oil
- 1 large eggplant, roughly diced
- 1 pound firm tofu, cut into 1-inch cubes, marinated in reduced sodium soy sauce
- 6 leaves kale, rinsed, destemmed, and roughly chopped
- ¾ cup Roasted Garlic Vinaigrette
- 3 cups warm Coconut Brown Rice (recipe follows)
- 3 cups warm Field Pea Curry (recipe follows)

**Make the Roasted Garlic Vinaigrette:** In a small saucepan over medium-high heat, heat 2 tablespoons oil. Sauté garlic for 2 minutes or until golden brown. Remove garlic from the oil with a slotted spoon and set aside to cool. Combine remaining oil, roasted garlic, and the rest of the ingredients (shallot through sesame oil) into a blender and whip together on high. Refrigerate for up to 3 days.

**Prepare the Eggplant + Tofu Salad:** In a large sauté pan, heat oil until it smokes. Carefully add the eggplant and tofu to the pan and fry for 5-10 minutes, until golden brown. Toss in the kale and cook for an additional 2 minutes. Fold in the vinaigrette and keep warm.

To serve, place ½ cup Coconut Brown Rice into each bowl followed by ½ cup Field Pea Curry. Top with the warm eggplant and tofu salad. Serve immediately.

**PER SERVING:** 560 calories, 39 grams fat, 8 grams saturated fat, 400 mg sodium, 45 grams carbohydrate (39 grams net carbs), 6 grams fiber, 10 grams sugar (0 added sugar), 13 grams protein

**VEGAN**

## Nutrition Bite

Eggplant is rich in an antioxidant called nasulin, which is linked to better brain health, reduced risk of cancer, and healthier joints. It's concentrated in the skin, so peeled eggplant won't have the same benefits.

## COCONUT BROWN RICE
**Makes approximately 3 cups**

14 ounces canned unsweetened coconut milk
1-inch ginger root, sliced in half
¾ stalk lemongrass, crushed, divided
1 tablespoon red pepper flakes

1 cup Louisiana brown rice, uncooked
1¼ cups coconut water
¾ cup water
½-inch ginger root, cut into thick rounds
¼ teaspoon sea salt

Place first 2 ingredients into a small pot with ½ stalk lemongrass and bring to a simmer. Immediately remove from heat and let steep for an hour to create a rice wash. Strain and and reserve liquid.

Place remaining 6 ingredients in a rice cooker with remaining lemongrass. When cooked, fluff with a fork and fold in ½ cup rice wash.

## FIELD PEA CURRY
**Makes 3-4 cups**

2 tablespoons light olive oil
½ stick cinnamon
¼ cup finely sliced fresh cilantro
½ yellow onion, diced
2 tablespoons brown curry powder (recipe follows)
1 tablespoon minced ginger
1 tablespoon minced garlic

½ cup field peas, uncooked (substitute black-eyed peas)
⅛ stalk lemongrass, beaten with the back of a wooden spoon or mallet
1 quart unsalted vegetable stock
2 tablespoons seasoned rice wine vinegar
1 tablespoon Sambal chili paste

In a large pot over medium-high heat, add oil and toast cinnamon stick for 5 minutes. Add cilantro and onion and sweat for 5 minutes, until translucent. Mix in brown curry powder, ginger, and garlic and sweat for an additional 3 minutes. Add peas, lemongrass, and vegetable stock and simmer uncovered until peas are tender, adding more stock as needed. Remove cinnamon stick and lemongrass, then add rice wine vinegar and sambal to the curry. Peas should be slightly overcooked. Smash when done.

## BROWN CURRY POWDER

**Makes 1½ cups**

**1 cup coriander seeds**
**½ teaspoon ground cloves**
**1 teaspoon allspice**
**2 tablespoons cumin**
**2 pods star anise (or 2 teaspoons Chinese Five Spice)**
**2 dried Thai chili peppers**
**1 cinnamon stick**
**1 tablespoon ground black cardamom**

Combine all spices in a small, heavy pan (we prefer cast iron) over medium heat. Stir constantly, until fragrant, taking care not to burn. Once toasted, transfer the spices to a bowl. Allow to cool, then grind in a spice grinder or with mortar and pestle. Sift out larger chunks and discard.

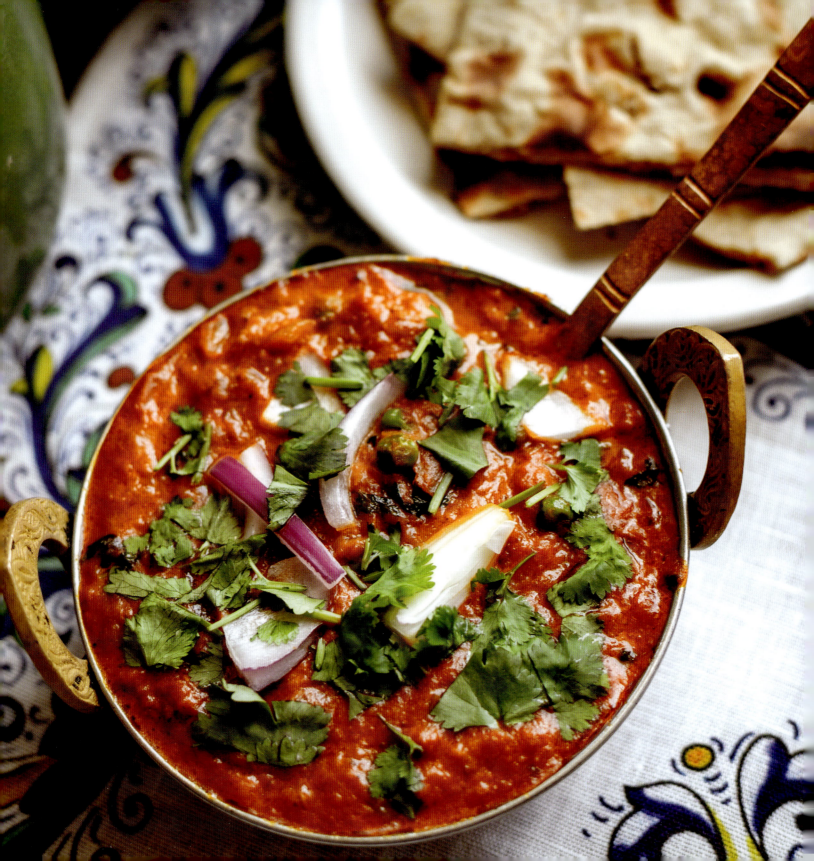

# Baingan Bharta
*Taste of India*

**Makes 2 servings**

*Baingan* is Hindi for "eggplant," and the literal translation of *bharta* is "mashed." But this isn't just any mashed eggplant. A signature of Taste of India in Monroe, our very first Indian Eat Fit partner restaurant, this savory dish is an explosion of flavor that you'll want to add to your regular culinary rotation.

- 1 eggplant
- 2 tablespoons extra virgin olive oil
- ½ tablespoon cumin seeds
- 2 garlic cloves
- 1 cinnamon stick
- 2 bay leaves
- ¼ cup onion, chopped
- 1 tablespoon Ginger Garlic Paste (recipe follows)
- ½ tablespoon turmeric powder
- ½ teaspoon salt
- ½ teaspoon chili powder
- ½ teaspoon cumin powder
- ½ tablespoon ground coriander
- ½ teaspoon garam masala
- 1 fresh tomato, chopped
- Fresh cilantro, for garnish

Preheat oven to 350 degrees. Wash eggplant and place in roasting pan. Brush skin with a tablespoon of olive oil and roast for 30-40 minutes, until soft enough to pierce with a fork. Let cool, then remove skin.

In a large skillet over medium heat, add a tablespoon of olive oil, then add cumin seeds, garlic cloves, cinnamon stick, and bay leaves, stirring until spices are well combined with oil.

Add onion and sauté until golden, approximately 4-5 minutes. Add Ginger Garlic Paste and turmeric and sauté another 2-3 minutes, until the strong garlic aroma has mellowed.

Finely chop or mash the roasted eggplant and add to pan. Add salt, chili powder, cumin powder, ground coriander, and garam masala, stirring until well-combined. Stir in chopped tomato and crush to release juices; finish by cooking for another 5 minutes, tasting and adjusting seasonings as needed. Remove bay leaves and cinnamon stick. Top with fresh cilantro and serve in a bowl, family style.

**PER SERVING:** 240 calories, 15 grams fat, 2 grams saturated fat, 620 mg sodium, 26 grams carbohydrate (15 grams net carbs), 11 grams fiber, 12 grams sugar (0 added sugar), 5 grams protein

GF, Vegan

## GINGER GARLIC PASTE

**Makes approximately 1 cup**

- 4 ounces fresh ginger, peeled
- 4 ounces garlic cloves, peeled
- 1 tablespoon extra virgin olive oil

Add ingredients to a food processor. Blend on high until smooth and light in color (occasionally stopping to scrape the sides). Store in the refrigerator in an airtight glass container for up to 6 months.

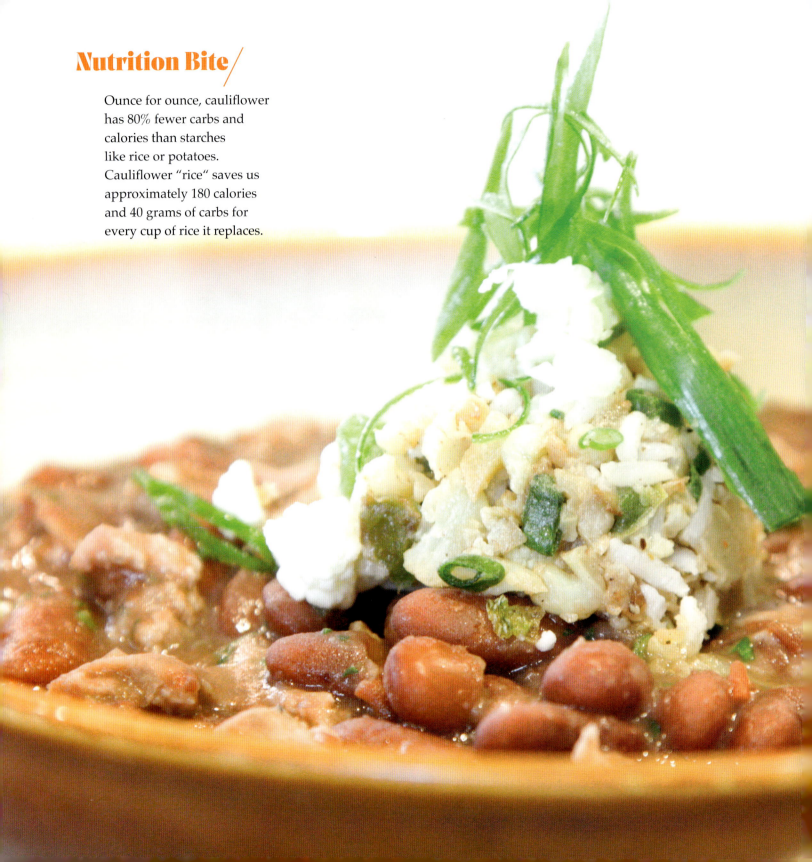

## Nutrition Bite

Ounce for ounce, cauliflower has 80% fewer carbs and calories than starches like rice or potatoes. Cauliflower "rice" saves us approximately 180 calories and 40 grams of carbs for every cup of rice it replaces.

# Red Beans + Cauliflower Rice
## *Curio*

**Makes 6 servings**

Cauliflower . . . we just can't get enough! It's no surprise when you take a look at its impressive credentials. Cauliflower is a culinary chameleon that can pose as everything from potatoes and grits to taco shells and pizza crust.

### Red Beans

- ½ pound dry red beans, soaked
- ½ small onion, diced
- ½ green bell pepper, diced
- 1 teaspoon chopped garlic
- 1 teaspoon chopped fresh thyme
- 6 cups unsalted chicken stock
- 4 ounces reduced sodium smoked turkey sausage, sliced
- ½ teaspoon sea salt
- ¼ teaspoon ground black pepper
- 2 tablespoons sliced green onion
- 1 tablespoon parsley, chopped

### Cauliflower Rice

- 2 cauliflower heads, cut into small florets
- 1½ tablespoons olive oil
- 1 small onion, finely diced
- ½ teaspoon sea salt
- ¼ cup water
- 2 tablespoons sliced green onion

**Cook the Red Beans:** Soak beans overnight, drain, and rinse. Place red beans, onion, bell pepper, garlic, and thyme in a large pot. Add chicken stock and bring to a boil. Reduce heat and simmer for 1 hour, stirring occasionally to prevent sticking.

Once beans are soft, remove a quarter of the beans. Puree with immersion blender or food processor and return to pot. Add smoked turkey sausage and cook an additional 30 minutes to an hour, until thickened. Add salt, pepper, green onion, and parsley then remove from heat. Serve over warm cauliflower rice.

**While the Red Beans are cooking, prepare the Cauliflower Rice:** Trim the cauliflower head, cutting away as much stem as possible. In batches, break up florets in a food processor and pulse until mixture is about the size of rice (don't overdo it or you'll end up with something more along the lines of cauliflower grits or mashed potatoes).

Heat oil in a large skillet over medium-high heat. Sauté onion until golden brown. Add cauliflower and salt and stir to combine. Add water and steam until cauliflower softens, about 5-7 minutes. Remove from heat and stir in green onion. Serve warm with red beans.

**PER SERVING:** 230 calories, 8 grams fat, 2 grams saturated fat, 450 mg sodium, 28 grams carbohydrate (19 grams net carbs), 9 grams fiber, 7 grams sugar (0 added sugar), 17 grams protein

GF

## By the Way

As a rice substitute, cauliflower doesn't even need to be cooked. Pulse it a few times in a food processor or use an old-fashioned cheese grater to crumble it into "rice" and you're ready to roll.

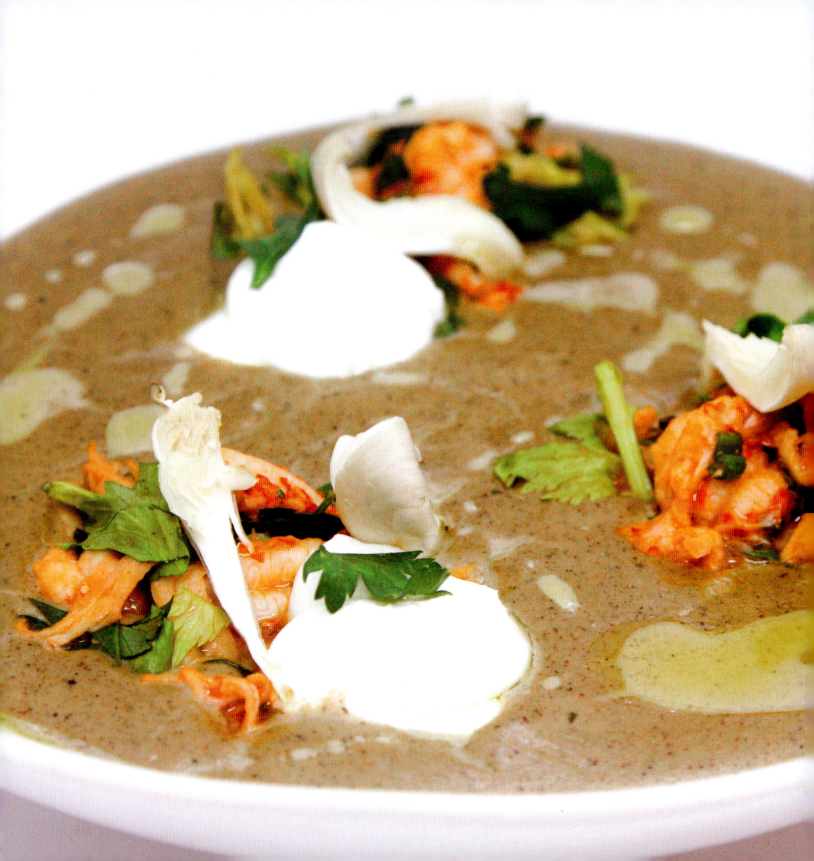

# Crawfish Mushroom + Goat Cheese Bisque
## Chef Carl Schaubhut

**Makes 12 servings**

"As chefs, our focus is all about taking care of others, making sure they love the food and love their experience. But as a chef, it's also part of our duty to nourish, ourselves included, from the inside out. This crawfish bisque makes it easy to do both." —Chef Carl

- 1 tablespoon olive oil
- 2 carrots, peeled and diced
- 2 onions, peeled and diced
- 1 rib celery, diced
- 2 cloves garlic, minced
- 1 teaspoon sea salt
- ½ teaspoon freshly ground black pepper
- ½ teaspoon dried oregano
- ½ teaspoon dried thyme
- 1 pound portobello mushrooms, diced (stems reserved)
- 1 pound crimini mushrooms, diced (or substitute baby Portobellos) (stems reserved)
- 1 batch Mushroom Stock (recipe follows)
- ½ teaspoon freshly ground black pepper
- 1 pound crawfish tails, rinsed
- 10 ounces goat cheese, divided
- 2 tablespoons chopped fresh basil
- 2 tablespoons chopped fresh thyme
- 2 tablespoons chopped fresh parsley
- 2 tablespoons lemon juice or white wine vinegar
- Truffle oil (optional)

In a large pot, heat oil over medium heat. Add carrots, onions, celery, garlic, salt, pepper, oregano, and thyme. Cook down for 15-20 minutes, stirring occasionally, until liquid starts to form and carrots are soft. Fold in mushrooms and cook for 10 minutes, stirring occasionally. Add Mushroom Stock. Bring to a boil then reduce heat to a simmer. Simmer for 30 minutes. Puree with an immersion blender until smooth. Return to a simmer, then fold in in crawfish tails, half of the goat cheese, and fresh herbs. Stir in lemon juice or vinegar.

Transfer to serving bowls. Garnish each bowl with goat cheese crumbles and a drop of truffle oil (if desired). Serve warm.

**PER SERVING:** 140 calories, 5 grams fat, 2.5 grams saturated fat, 270 mg sodium, 14 grams carbohydrate (11 grams net carbs), 3 grams fiber, 6 grams sugar (0 added sugar), 13 grams protein
**GF**

## Make It Meatless

Make it vegetarian with tofu (firm and cubed) or cooked white beans in place of crawfish tails. Use dairy-free cream cheese in place of goat cheese to take it all the way vegan.

## Tip

You can usually use dried herbs in place of fresh and vice versa, just use ⅓ of the amount of dried herbs as you would fresh (or 3 times the amount of fresh as you would dried).

## MUSHROOM STOCK

### Makes approximately 3 quarts

1 gallon water
Reserved mushroom stems
1 onion, cut into large dice
1 head celery, cut into large dice
3 carrots, cut into large dice
1 bay leave
1 handful fresh thyme

In a large pot, add all ingredients and bring to boil. Reduce heat and simmer for 30 minutes and strain. Reserve for bisque or freeze for future use.

## Time Saver /

Use 3 quarts store-bought unsalted vegetable stock in place of the homemade mushroom stock.

# Salt Swaps

Salt isn't all bad. In fact, we all need it, at least to some degree, for healthy nerves, muscle contraction, and blood volume. And some of us actually need to add *more* into our diets. But unless you're an athlete losing buckets of sweat, a construction worker outside in the heat, or you just generally live, work, and play in a hot, humid environment, it's probably a good idea to be mindful of your sodium intake. Too much can up our odds of high blood pressure, bloating, and fluid retention, among other health issues.

Whether it's sea salt, Kosher salt, or regular old table salt, ounce-for-ounce, the sodium content is essentially the same. But coarse, larger-grain salts give us the *perception* of more salt. Since the larger grains don't pack together as tightly, coarser salts have a slightly lower sodium content per spoonful (about 480 mg per ¼ teaspoon compared to 590 mg for the same amount of finely ground salt).

**CAJUN SEASONING**  Switch from traditional Creole Seasoning (350 mg per ¼ teaspoon) to Chef Paul Prudhomme's Magic Seasoning Blends (average 100 mg per ¼ teaspoon).

**HOT SAUCE**  Switch from Louisiana Hot Sauce (240 mg per teaspoon) to Tabasco (just 35 mg sodium per teaspoon).

**CHEESE**  Make the switch from feta (330 mg per ounce) to goat cheese (80 mg per ounce) or from cheddar (180 mg per ounce) to Swiss (65 mg per ounce).

**PASTA SAUCE**  Switch from regular pasta sauce (400+ mg per ½ cup) to Sal & Judy's Heart Smart sauce (135 mg per ½ cup).

## "Salt-Less" Strategies

Gradually use less salt to give your taste buds time to acclimate. Experiment with herbs, spices, and vinegars in place of salt. Add salt last, not during cooking.

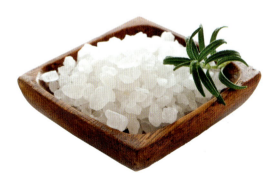

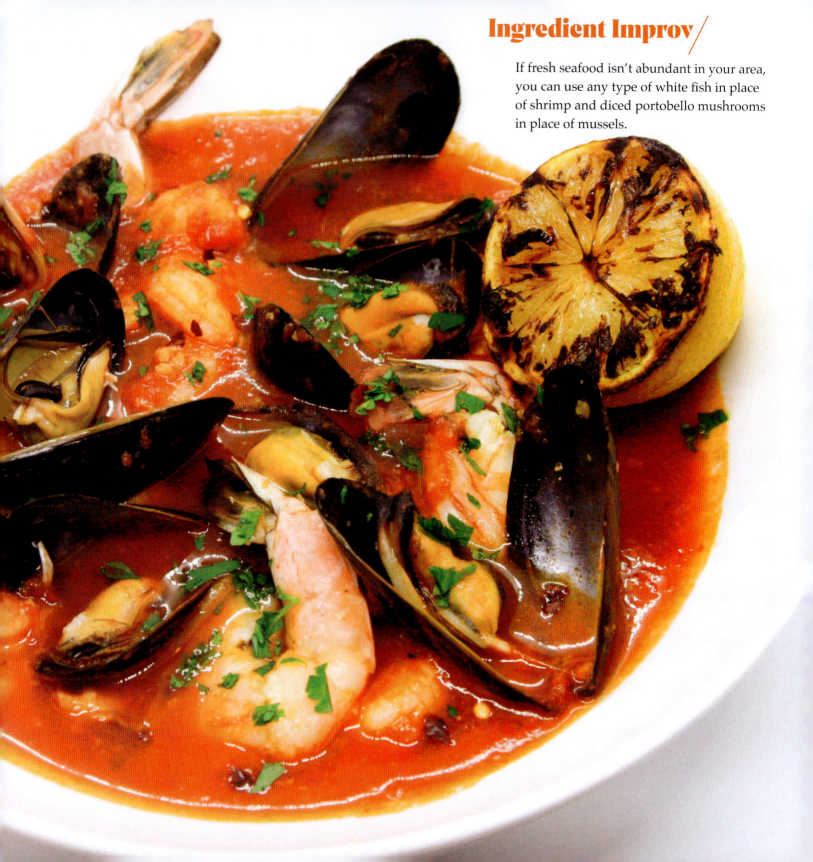

## Ingredient Improv/

If fresh seafood isn't abundant in your area, you can use any type of white fish in place of shrimp and diced portobello mushrooms in place of mussels.

# Seafood Cioppino
## Tommy's Cuisine

**Makes 8 servings**

Talk about a meal that can multitask! In addition to creating this tasty dish tonight, you can repurpose leftovers to add protein to a green salad or make tacos on low-carb tortillas for lunch tomorrow. Add extra tomatoes to the cioppino sauce to drizzle over grilled chicken breasts, and you have dinner tomorrow night.

1½ pounds fresh fish, cubed (scraps reserved for stock)
1 pound jumbo shrimp, peeled (shells reserved for stock)
¼ teaspoon sea salt
½ teaspoon freshly ground black pepper
4 tablespoons extra virgin olive oil
½ cup chopped fennel bulb
½ cup chopped shallots
6 garlic cloves, chopped
1 pound fresh mussels
1 batch Seafood Tomato Stock (recipe follows)
½ teaspoon sea salt
1 lemon, halved

Season fish and shrimp on both sides with salt and pepper. In a sauté pan, heat olive oil. Add fennel and shallots and sweat for 2 minutes, then toast the chopped garlic. Place the fish and shrimp into the pan, being careful not to splash the oil. Sear the seafood slightly on both sides, but do not cook all the way through.

Add mussels, Seafood Tomato Stock, and salt to the seared seafood. Bring to a low simmer and cover. Steam mussels for 90 seconds. Once the mussels have opened, taste the broth for seasoning. Add a squeeze of lemon. Serve hot.

### SEAFOOD TOMATO STOCK

**Makes 1½ cups**

Fish and shrimp trimmings
2 cups water
1 celery stalk, chopped
1 onion, chopped
1 tomato, chopped
Pinch of sea salt
Pinch of freshly ground black pepper

In a small soup pot, add water and reserved seafood shells and fish scraps. Add celery, onion, and tomato. Season with salt and pepper. Gently simmer—do not boil—for 45 minutes. Strain broth through a fine strainer. Reserve for cioppino or freeze for future use.

**PER SERVING:** 270 calories, 10 grams fat, 1.5 grams saturated fat, 430 mg sodium, 6 grams carbohydrate (6 grams net carbs), <1 gram fiber, 1 gram sugar (0 added sugar), 39 grams protein
GF, Low Carb

## Nutrition Bite /

Add chickpeas and tofu for more fiber and protein.

## Time Saver /

If making homemade stock isn't your thing, use 1 cup of store-bought seafood stock (unsalted vegetable stock will do in a pinch) blended with ½ cup of no-salt-added canned diced tomatoes.

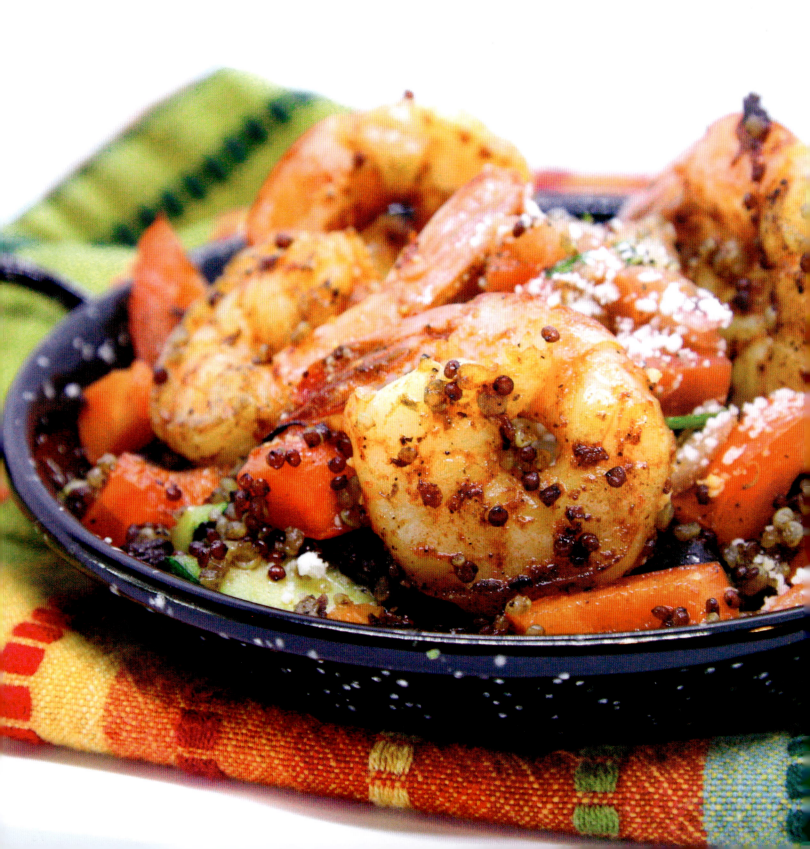

# Shrimp Quinoa Jambalaya
## Mestizo Louisiana Mexican Cuisine

**Makes 8 servings**

Quinoa is nutrient dense, offering an excellent source of both protein and fiber. But it's also calorie dense, cramming a lot of carbs and calories into a small serving. Jim Urdiales of Mestizo solves this issue by incorporating zucchini and squash into his quinoa jambalaya to replace some of the quinoa, saving us the carbs and calories.

2 tablespoons light olive oil
½ cup chipotle sauce (such as Tabasco Chipotle Pepper Sauce), divided
1 cup cubed zucchini
1 cup cubed squash
1 cup canned black beans, drained and rinsed
3 cups quinoa, cooked
Dash of sea salt
16 jumbo shrimp, peeled, with tail-on (or 1 cup of cubed tofu)

In a skillet over medium-high heat, heat olive oil, 6 tablespoons of chipotle sauce, zucchini, and squash and cook until soft. Mix in black beans, quinoa, and salt. Sauté for 3 minutes. Sauté shrimp (or tofu) separately with remaining chipotle sauce. Place on top of quinoa and serve warm.

**PER SERVING:** 170 calories, 5 grams fat, 0.5 gram saturated fat, 490 mg sodium, 23 grams carbohydrate (19 grams net carbs), 4 grams fiber, 1 gram sugar (0 added sugar), 11 grams protein
**GF**

## Make It Vegan

Serve with tofu in place of shrimp for a 100% plant-based jambalaya.

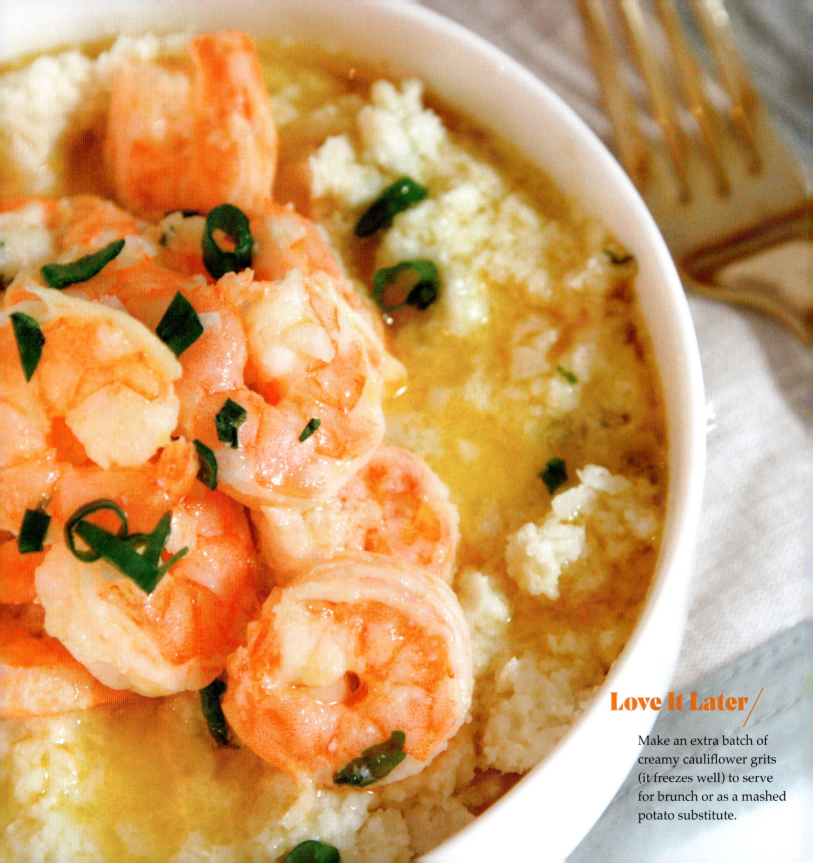

### Love It Later

Make an extra batch of creamy cauliflower grits (it freezes well) to serve for brunch or as a mashed potato substitute.

# Scampi-Style Shrimp + Creamy Cauliflower Grits

## Boulevard American Bistro

**Makes 4 servings**

You won't even recognize the cauliflower in this recipe. When we serve this dish, people often have no idea it's good for them. We do whatever it takes to support our own around here, even if it means doing it on the sly!

### For the Shrimp
½ cup extra virgin olive oil
3 garlic cloves, minced
¼ cup chopped fresh parsley
2 teaspoons chopped fresh rosemary
1 lemon, zested and juiced
½ teaspoon sea salt
½ teaspoon white pepper
1 pound jumbo shrimp, peeled

### For the Cauliflower Grits
1 large cauliflower head, cut into small florets
½ cup canned unsweetened coconut milk
2 tablespoons reduced fat cream cheese
½ teaspoon sea salt
½ teaspoon white pepper

**Prepare the Shrimp:** Preheat grill. In a medium bowl, combine olive oil, garlic, parsley, rosemary, lemon zest, salt, and pepper. Remove half of marinade to a separate bowl and set aside. Add shrimp to first bowl and coat with olive oil mixture. Add lemon juice and toss to mix. Refrigerate for 30 minutes.

**While the Shrimp are marinating, prepare the Cauliflower Grits:** In batches, pulse cauliflower in a food processor until florets break down into fine, grain-like pieces. In a large saucepan over medium heat, warm coconut milk. Add cauliflower and cook until soft. Add more milk if needed. Fold in cream cheese and stir until melted. Season with salt and pepper and set aside while you grill the shrimp.

Place shrimp onto grill and cook 2-3 minutes on each side, basting with marinade throughout. Cook until shrimp are opaque.

Heat the reserved marinade. Serve grilled shrimp over warm cauliflower grits drizzled with 1 tablespoon of reserved marinade.

**PER SERVING:** 460 calories, 35 grams fat, 9 grams saturated fat, 560 mg sodium, 14 grams carbohydrate (9 grams net carbs), 5 grams fiber, 5 grams sugar (0 added sugar), 28 grams protein
GF, Low Carb

## Tip/
This recipe calls for culinary coconut milk—the type that's in the can, not the refrigerated section. Look for brands with a clean, simple ingredient list. We like Thai Kitchen's Unsweetened Coconut Milk.

## Time Saver/
For an easy shortcut, use store-bought cauliflower "rice." Look for it in the produce section or freezer aisle.

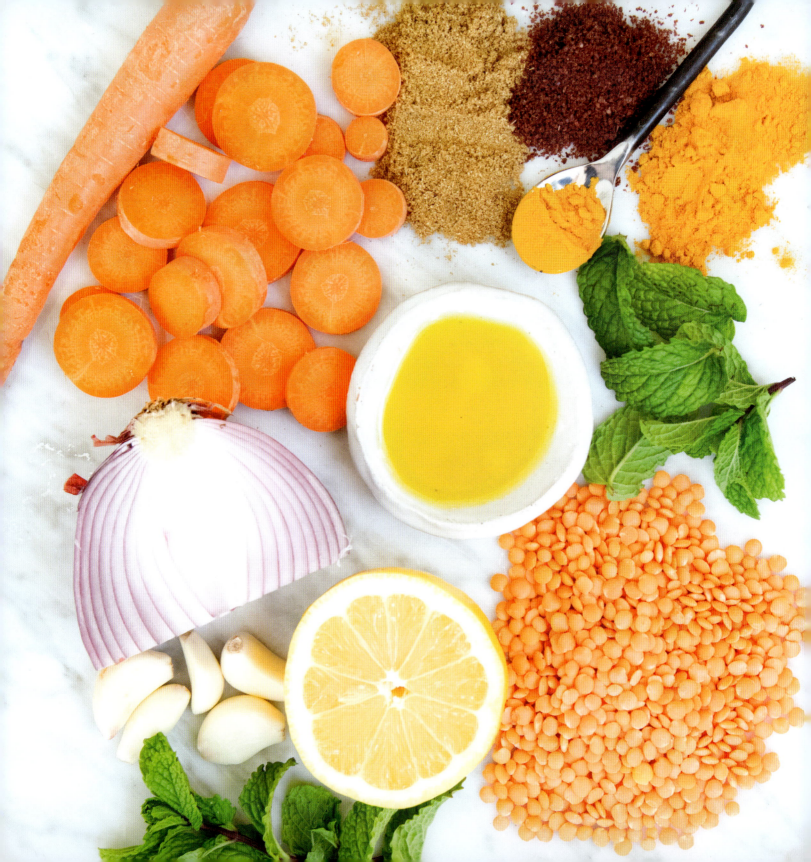

# Mediterranean Whole Lentil Soup
## Attiki Bar & Grill

**Makes 4 servings**

Traditionally, this soup calls for pureed lentils, but the sodium in Attiki's original version was too high for Eat Fit. Now, Attiki removes a batch of the lentil soup before salting—and before pureeing—creating an Eat Fit version with whole lentils. This soup is vegan, protein rich, and full of fiber. It is also hearty enough to serve as an entrée.

- 1½ cups whole red lentils, rinsed
- 4 cups water (at room temperature)
- ½ tablespoon extra virgin olive oil
- ¼ large red onion, diced
- ¼ large carrot, diced
- ¾ tablespoon minced garlic
- ¾ tablespoon cumin
- ½ tablespoon turmeric
- 1 dash freshly ground black pepper
- 4 cups unsalted vegetable broth
- ¾ teaspoon sea salt
- 2 tablespoons lemon juice
- Fresh mint for garnish
- Sumac for garnish

In a medium pot, soak lentils in water for 30 minutes. Bring lentils to a boil after soaking (this helps to reduce cooking time). Drain and set aside.

In a large pot over medium heat, add oil and sauté onion and carrot for 7-10 minutes, until soft. Add garlic, cumin, turmeric, and black pepper and sauté for 2 minutes. Stir in lentils and broth and bring to a boil. Reduce heat, cover, and simmer for 1 hour, or until lentils are softened.

Mix in salt and lemon juice and let sit for 5 minutes. Serve hot, garnished with fresh mint and a dash of sumac.

**PER SERVING:** 310 calories, 3.5 grams fat, 0.5 grams saturated fat, 470 mg sodium, 54 grams carbohydrate (46 grams net carbs), 8 grams fiber, 5 grams sugar (0 added sugar), 18 grams protein

GF, Vegan

> *"I love to cook, and I love to feed. This soup is inspired by the flavors of my Mediterranean childhood, seasoned with sumac's savory tart and lemony spice."*
>
> —Diana Canahuati, owner of Attiki Bar & Grill

## By the Way

Attiki uses red lentils for this dish, but you can use any color in the lentil rainbow.

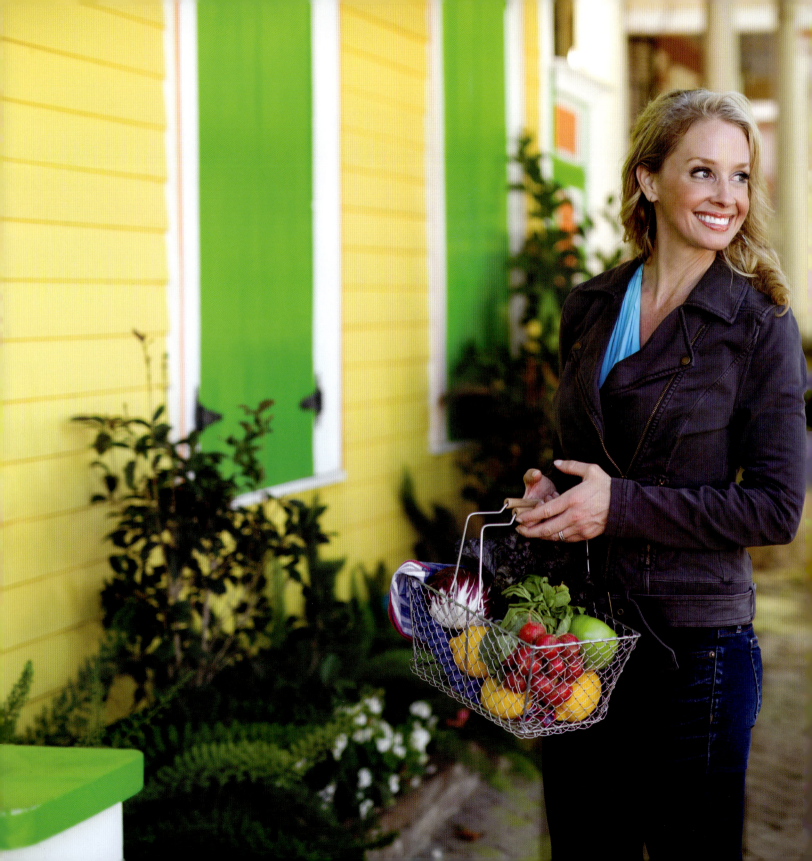

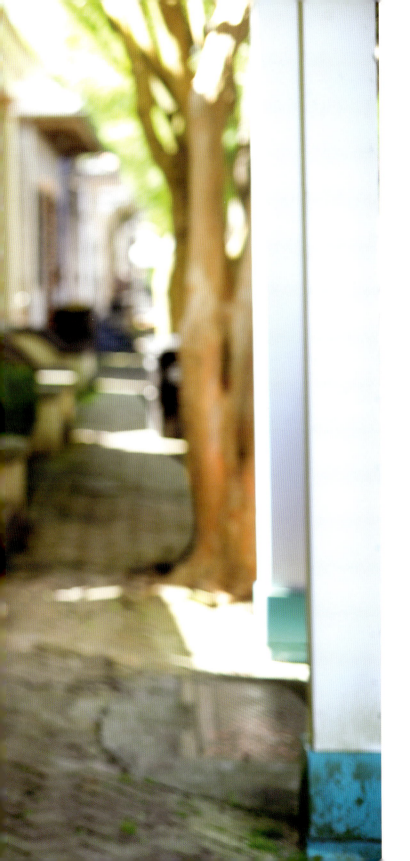

# 3
## CRISP
### *Starter Salads, Fruits + Foliage*

Set the scene for your next dinner party! Not only will these salads make a great first impression, they will also help set the tone for the whole meal. When we start our meals with clean, nutrient-dense foods, it is easier to curb our cravings for mindless nibbling.

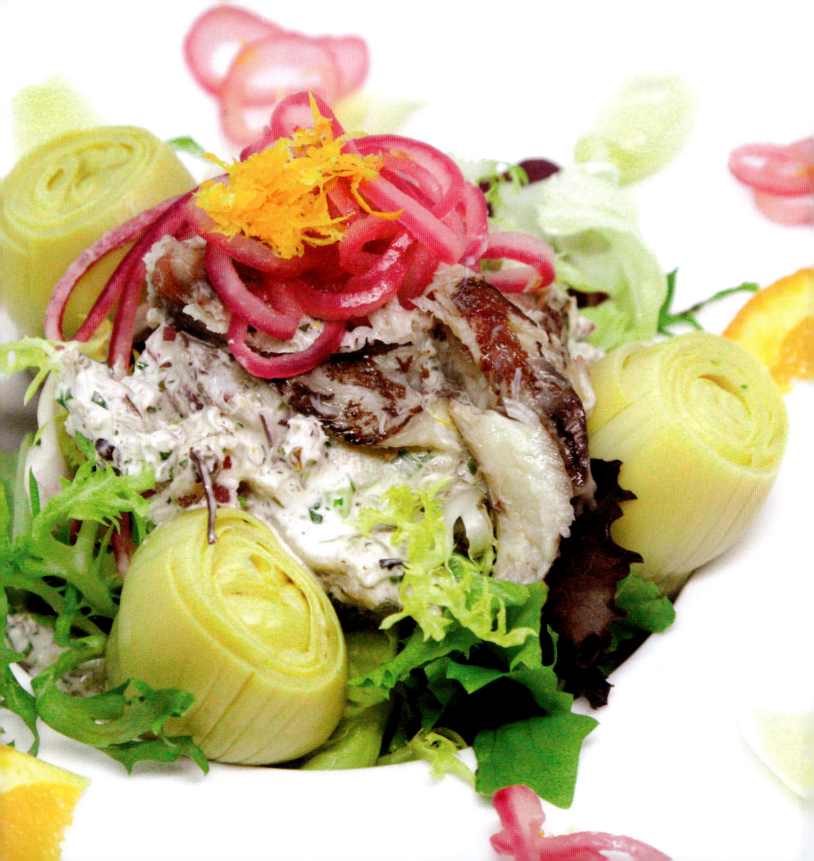

# Crabmeat + Artichoke Salad with Citrus Dressing
## Jacques-Imo's Café

**Makes 8 servings**

Self-proclaimed as the restaurant that serves "real Nawlins food," Jacques-Imo's is well known for its rich, unusual, over-the-top dishes. For years, diners have enjoyed menu items including alligator cheesecake and the deep-fried po' boy. However, in recent years, Chef Jacques has made wellness a top priority in his own life, creating an ever-increasing number of healthier dishes like this citrusy crabmeat salad, which Jacques-Imo's serves each year at French Quarter Fest.

⅔ cup Jacques-Imo's Citrus Dressing (recipe follows)
5 cups mixed field greens
½ pound lump crabmeat
1 pound crab claw meat
1½ cups Ravigote Sauce (page 183)
14-ounce can whole artichoke hearts, drained
1 orange, sliced
¼ cup Pickled Red Onions for garnish (page 163)

Combine Jacques-Imo's Citrus Dressing and mixed greens in a bowl. Toss to coat. In a separate bowl, very carefully fold crabmeat into Ravigote so as not to shred the crabmeat. Portion and plate the greens, then top with a heaping scoop of Ravigote. Garnish with artichoke hearts, orange slices, and Pickled Red Onions.

### JACQUES-IMO'S CITRUS DRESSING

**Makes approximately ⅔ cup**

⅓ cup light olive oil
2 tablespoons apple cider vinegar
2 tablespoons fresh lemon juice
2 tablespoons fresh orange juice
¼ teaspoon lemon zest
1 orange, zested
Pinch of sea salt
1 pinch freshly ground black pepper

Whisk together oil, vinegar, lemon juice, and orange juice. Add lemon zest, orange zest, salt, and pepper. Mix to combine.

**PER SERVING:** 300 calories, 19 grams fat, 3 grams saturated fat, 680 mg sodium, 15 grams carbohydrate (9 grams net carbs), 4 grams fiber, 6 grams sugar (0 added sugar), 19 grams protein
GF, Low Carb

## Sodium Check

Use frozen artichoke hearts in place of canned artichokes for a lower sodium option.

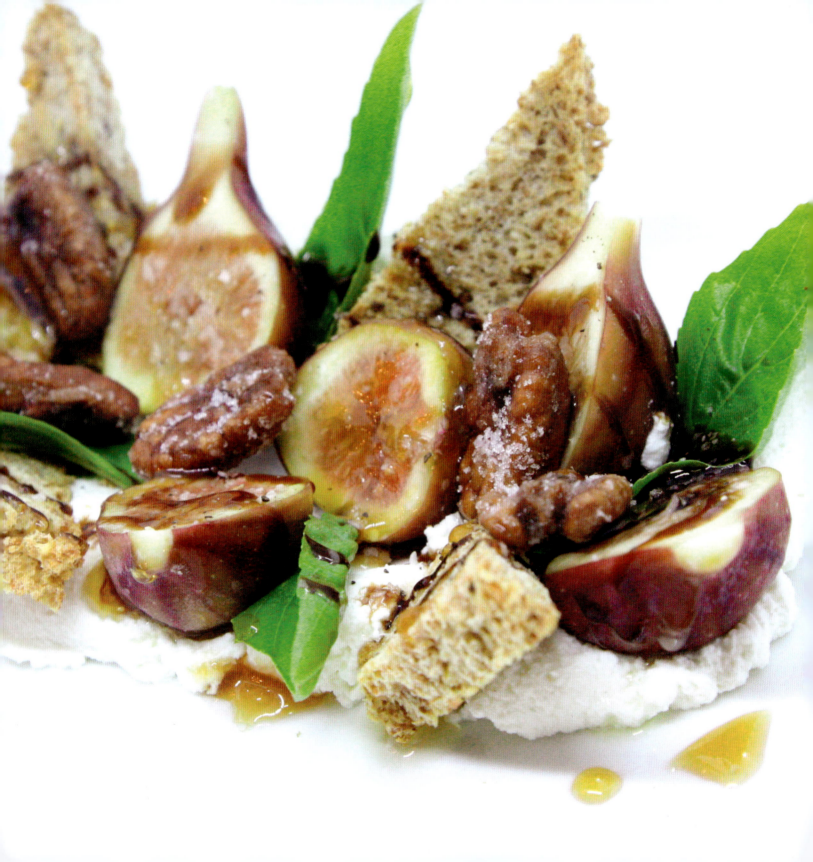

# Fig Street Fig Salad
## Ye Olde College Inn

**Makes 6 servings**

A local Uptown favorite, Ye Olde College Inn pairs figs and fresh basil from their farm across the street with local pecans and local honey. Their house-made croutons are reason enough to make this salad, adding a fantastically savory crunch. With a schmear of ricotta and a drizzle of balsamic glaze, this salad is fancy enough to serve for company yet simple enough for a weeknight staple.

- 2 slices whole grain bread, cut into ½-inch cubes
- 15 fresh figs, halved
- 2½ tablespoons extra virgin olive oil
- 2½ tablespoons balsamic glaze, divided
- ¼ teaspoon sea salt
- 1 pinch freshly ground black pepper
- 1½ cups part-skim ricotta cheese
- ⅓ cup toasted pecans
- 12 basil leaves
- 1 tablespoon honey

Preheat oven to 350 degrees. To make croutons, place the bread on a baking sheet and toast in the oven for 6-8 minutes until crispy.

Toss figs in oil and 1½ tablespoons balsamic glaze. Toss with salt and pepper and set aside. Schmear ricotta onto serving plates. Top with figs and garnish with pecans, croutons, basil, 1 tablespoon drizzle of balsamic glaze, and a dot of honey.

**PER SERVING:** 340 calories, 16 grams fat, 4.5 grams saturated fat, 210 mg sodium, 43 grams carbohydrate (37 grams net carbs), 6 grams fiber, 28 grams sugar (3 grams added sugar), 11 grams protein

VEGETARIAN

## Tip

You can find balsamic glaze in stores, but it's also super easy to make: simply bring 1 cup of balsamic vinegar to a boil then simmer until it is reduced to ¼ cup.

## Nutrition Bite

Ricotta is naturally low in sodium, saturated fat, and calories, yet it adds an element of creamy richness.

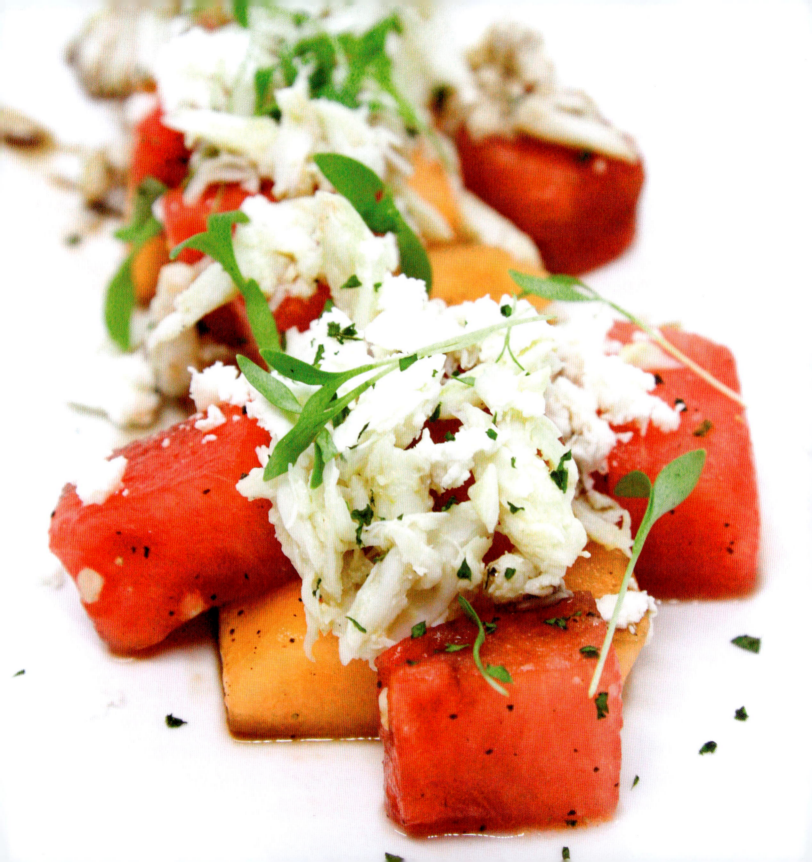

# Summer Melon Salad
## Ye Olde College Inn

**Makes 4 servings**

Sprinkle sea salt on a watermelon? Either you've done it already or you're about to be introduced to your new favorite summertime salad. It's refreshingly sweet, savory, and even slightly creamy. Sound too good to be true? That's what we thought until we tried it. This Summer Melon Salad is perfect for backyard cookouts, served as an appetizer, a side salad, or even as a family-style platter. Make extra to keep on hand as a nutritious, anytime snack.

½ cantaloupe, cut into 4 slices
2 cups watermelon, cut into 2-inch cubes
Pinch of sea salt
Pinch of freshly ground black pepper
8 ounces lump crabmeat
4 tablespoons goat cheese, crumbled
2 tablespoons balsamic vinegar
4 teaspoons extra virgin olive oil

On serving plates, divide cantaloupe slices and cubed watermelon. Sprinkle with salt and pepper. Top each serving with 2 ounces crabmeat and 1 tablespoon goat cheese. Drizzle with balsamic vinegar and oil. Serve chilled.

**PER SERVING:** 160 calories, 7 grams fat, 2 grams saturated fat, 260 mg sodium, 13 grams carbohydrate (12 grams net carbs), 1 gram fiber, 11 grams sugar (0 added sugar), 12 grams protein
**GF**

## Nutrition Bite

Ye Olde College Inn's original recipe called for feta, but we swapped it out for goat cheese. Ounce for ounce, goat cheese has 75% less sodium than its saltier cousin.

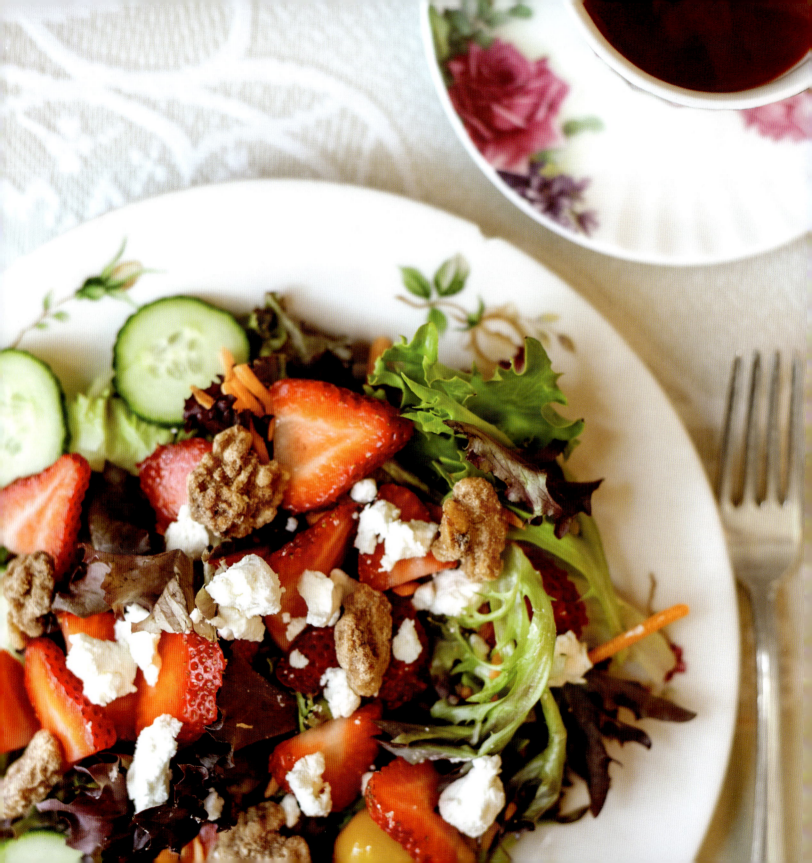

# Strawberry Fields Forever with Tea-Infused Berry Vinaigrette
## English Tea Room

**Makes 2 servings**

Tea-infused vinaigrette and Chef Diamonte's house-made candied walnuts are the stars of this show, with a strong supporting cast of beautiful fresh strawberries and creamy goat cheese.

**6 cups spring mix**
**1 cup strawberries, sliced**
**¼ cup candied walnuts (page 167)**
**¼ cup crumbled goat cheese**
**½ cup cherry tomatoes**
**½ cucumber, thinly sliced**
**2 tablespoons grated carrot**
**2 ounces tea-infused Berry Vinaigrette (page 178)**

In a large salad bowl, toss together spring mix, strawberries, candied walnuts, goat cheese, tomatoes, cucumber, and carrots. Divvy up onto two plates and serve with tea-infused Berry Vinaigrette.

**PER SERVING:** 260 calories, 19 grams fat, 5 grams saturated fat, 230 mg sodium, 22 grams carbohydrate (15 net carbs), 7 grams fiber, 9 grams sugar, 3 grams added sugar, 8 grams protein
**GF**

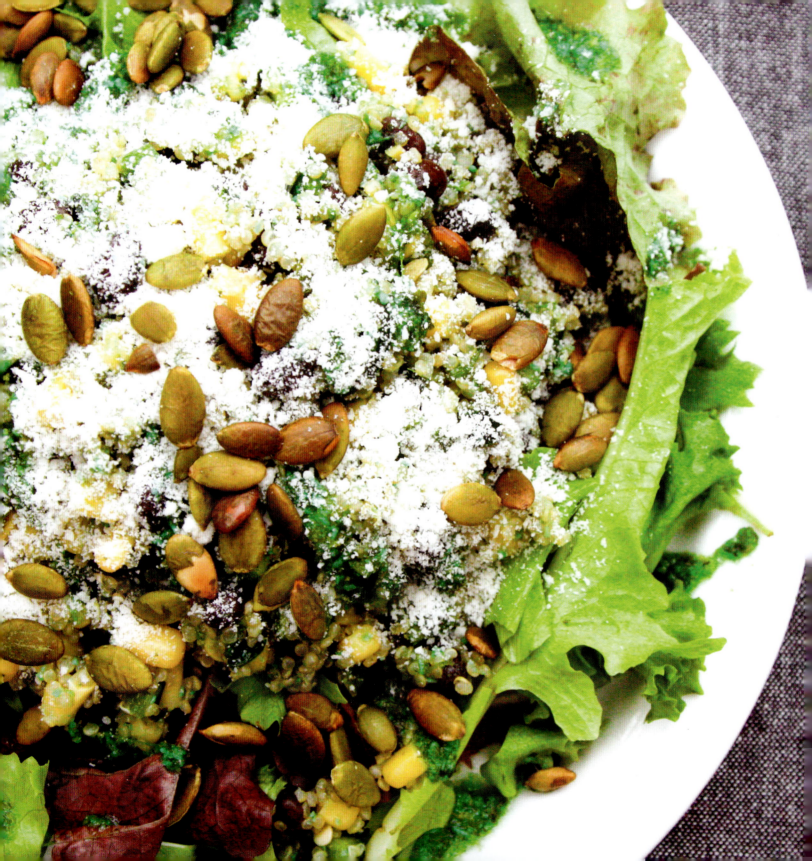

# Esmeralda Salad
## *Carmo*

**Makes 4 servings**

Plant based with the option for vegan, but hearty and filling. We promise, you'll feel good after you eat it.

- 4 cups cooked quinoa
- ¼ cup cooked black beans (or canned, drained, and rinsed)
- ¼ cup organic sweet corn kernels
- ¼ cup chopped cilantro
- ¼ cup chopped poblano peppers
- ⅓ cup + 4 tablespoons Esmeralda Dressing (recipe follows)
- 4 cups mixed salad greens
- ¼ cup cotija or vegan Parmesan cheese
- ¼ cup toasted pumpkin seeds

Toss quinoa, black beans, sweet corn, cilantro, and poblano with ⅓ cup prepared Esmeralda Dressing. On a large platter (or individual salad plates), evenly spread spring mix. Spoon quinoa-black bean mixture over the lettuce, creating a peak in the middle of the plate. Sprinkle cheese and pumpkin seeds on top. Drizzle 1 tablespoon dressing over each portion and serve immediately.

### ESMERALDA DRESSING

**Makes approximately 1 cup**

- 1 ripe (bright green) Anaheim pepper, seeded and roughly chopped
- ½ Serrano pepper, seeded and roughly chopped
- ¼ teaspoon toasted ground cumin
- ¼ teaspoon toasted ground coriander
- ¼ cup unsweetened coconut flakes
- ½ cup sushi rice wine vinegar
- ¼ teaspoon sea salt

Blend all ingredients together in a food processor until a thick but pourable mixture forms. Add a little extra rice wine vinegar if needed.

**PER SERVING:** 370 calories, 11 grams fat, 4 grams saturated fat, 560 mg sodium, 55 grams carbohydrate (46 grams net carbs), 9 grams fiber, 8 grams sugar (0 added sugar), 15 grams protein

GF, VEGETARIAN

## Note

Cotija cheese tastes like a cross between feta and Parmesan and can be found at most Latin markets.

## Toasting Spices

Toasting spices intensifies their flavor. It's best to toast them whole before grinding, but ground spices can also be toasted. Put the spices in a small, heavy pan (we prefer cast iron) over medium heat. Stir constantly, until fragrant, taking care not to burn. Once toasted, immediately transfer the spices to a bowl or parchment paper and gently stir or spread around to stop the cooking.

## Serve It Up

Carmo serves this salad chilled, but we also love lightly roasting the quinoa, beans, and corn first.

# Griddled Summer Squash and Tender Greens
## Commander's Palace

**Makes 4 servings**

In spite of the name, this dish can be made with so many different vegetables, depending on what's in season: golden beets, cauliflower, Brussels sprouts—as long as you like it, anything goes.

2 large or 4 small yellow summer squash or zucchini
1 pinch kosher salt
1 pinch freshly ground black pepper
1 teaspoon coconut oil
¼ red onion
6 ounces mixed greens, such as arugula and baby kale
2 tablespoons Steen's Cane Vinaigrette (page 179)

Wash squash and pat dry. Cut in half lengthwise, then cut into quarter-inch thick half-moons or rounds. Season with salt and pepper. In a skillet over medium-high heat, sauté squash in coconut oil. Cook until caramelized on outside, but still firm.

Clean and remove root and skin of quarter of a red onion. Slice thin. Rinse under cold water to lessen astringency. Prepare salad of greens, squash, and onion. Toss and drizzle with Steen's Cane Vinaigrette.

**PER SERVING:** 50 calories, 2 grams fat, 0.5 gram saturated fat, 150 mg sodium, 8 grams carbohydrate (6 grams net carbs), 2 grams fiber, 4 grams sugar (0 added sugar), 2 grams protein
GF, Low Carb, Vegan

# Avocado Salad
## Cleo's Mediterranean Cuisine & Grocery

**Makes 4 servings**

This salad is one of my personal favorites and the reason I fell in love with Cleo's. I love to add grilled shrimp; it's the perfect accompaniment to this fresh, hearty salad. Garnished beautifully with pomegranate and pumpkin seeds, Cleo's avocado salad is as beautiful as it is delicious.

- 4 cups spring mix
- 1 avocado, diced
- 2 tablespoons lemon juice
- 4 tablespoons toasted pumpkin seeds
- 1 teaspoon Cleo's House Seasoning Blend (recipe follows)
- 4 tablespoons Cleo's Lemon Dressing (page 172)
- 4 tablespoons pomegranate seeds
- 1 banana pepper, sliced into rings
- ¼ cup radish slices, shaved thin

Plate the spring mix. Top spring mix with avocado and drizzle with lemon juice. Top with pumpkin seeds and a dash of Cleo's House Seasoning Blend. Drizzle each salad with 1 tablespoon of Cleo's Lemon Dressing and garnish with pomegranate seeds, banana pepper rings, and shaved radish. Serve immediately.

### CLEO'S HOUSE SEASONING BLEND

**Makes approximately ¾ cup**

- ½ teaspoon sea salt
- ½ teaspoon freshly ground black pepper
- ½ teaspoon ground cumin
- ½ teaspoon coriander seed
- ½ teaspoon curry powder
- ½ teaspoon paprika
- ⅛ cup minced garlic
- ½ teaspoon onion powder
- ½ teaspoon dried oregano
- ½ teaspoon chili powder
- ¼ teaspoon black sesame seeds

Mix all ingredients together and store in an air-tight container.

**PER SERVING:** 180 calories, 14 grams fat, 2 grams saturated fat, 150 mg sodium, 12 grams carbohydrate (6 grams net carbs), 6 grams fiber, 3 grams sugar (0 added sugar), 3 grams protein

GF, Low Carb, Vegan

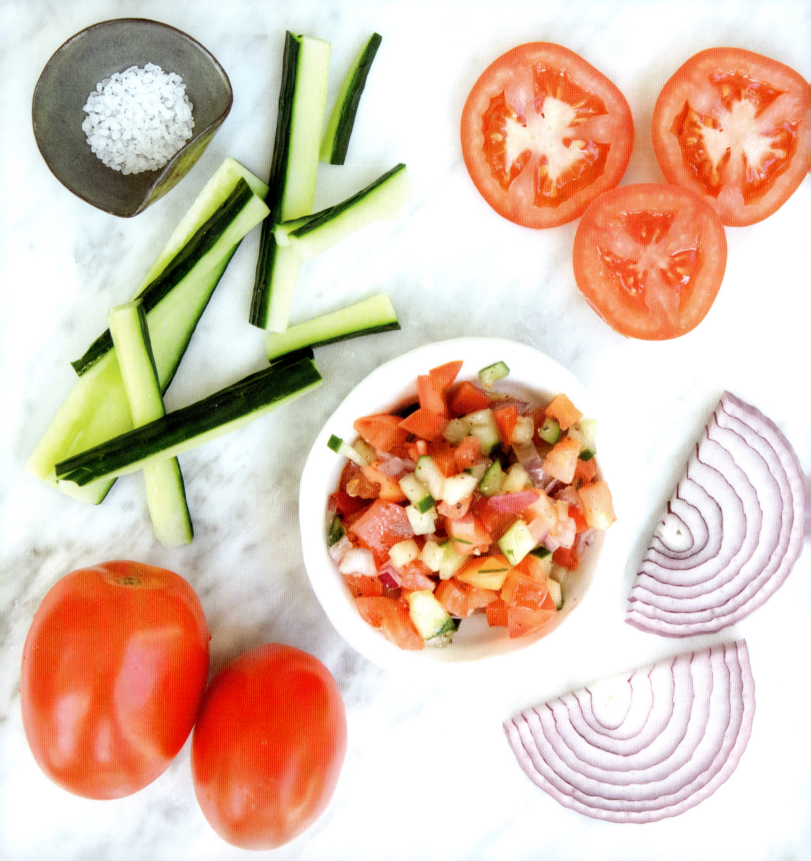

# Chopped Mediterranean Salad

*Attiki Bar & Grill*

**Makes 1½ cups**

Attiki's spices and fresh herbs give this unassuming little salad a virtual explosion of flavors.

2 Roma tomatoes, diced
1 small cucumber, diced
¼ medium red onion, diced
¼ cup chopped fresh parsley
1 tablespoon chopped fresh mint
1 tablespoon extra virgin olive oil
2 tablespoons lemon juice
2 teaspoons sumac
¼ teaspoon freshly ground black pepper
⅛ teaspoon sea salt

In a large bowl, combine all ingredients and toss until evenly mixed. Serve immediately or chill before serving.

**PER SERVING (¼ CUP):** 40 calories, 2.5 grams fat, 0 saturated fat, 25 mg sodium, 4 grams carbohydrate (3 grams net carbs), 1 gram fiber, 2 grams sugar (0 added sugar), <1 gram protein
GF, Low Carb, Vegan, Low Sodium

## Love It Later /

Leftovers pull triple duty as a topping for lean protein, a garnish for salads, or a playful twist on pico de gallo.

## su * mac /

Sumac is a Middle Eastern spice known for its versatility and tangy, lemon flavor.

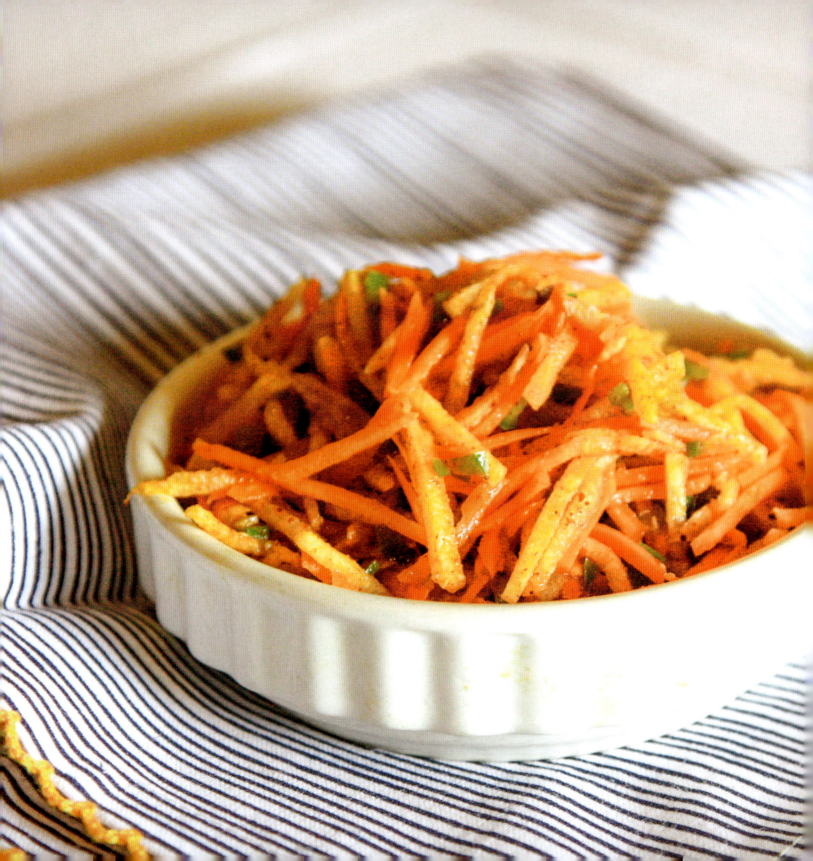

# Jicama Slaw
## Café Vermilionville

**Makes 4 servings**

Slaw doesn't have to be a mayo-drenched event. This jicama slaw is clean, crunchy, and bursting with flavor. It works well as a starter, a side dish, or as a topping for pretty much any main dish.

½ jicama or 1 Granny Smith apple, skin-on, cut into matchstick slices
1 carrot, julienned
1 jalapeño, thinly sliced
1 teaspoon chili powder
1 teaspoon red pepper flakes
¼ teaspoon sea salt
1 teaspoon freshly ground pepper
1 teaspoon Swerve Granular
¼ cup extra virgin olive oil
¼ cup rice wine vinegar

In a medium bowl, combine sliced jicama, carrot, jalapeño, chili powder, red pepper flakes, salt, pepper, and Swerve. Add olive oil and rice wine vinegar. Soak for at least 1 hour. Serve with a slotted spoon to drain excess liquid. Refrigerate for up to 3 days.

**PER SERVING:** 170 calories, 14 grams fat, 2 grams saturated fat, 150 mg sodium, 12 grams carbohydrate (7 grams net carbs), 5 grams fiber, 3 grams sugar (0 added sugar), <1 gram protein
GF, Low Carb, Vegan

## ji * ca * ma

Jicama is a crisp, white-fleshed root vegetable with the texture of an apple but without the sweetness. Remove the outer, bark-like skin to find the juicy, crunchy flesh inside. If you can't find it at your local grocery or farmer's market, use green apples as a jicama stand-in.

## Ingredient Improv

Regular sugar can be used in place of Swerve. This recipe calls for only 1 teaspoon, spread over 4 servings, so it's not enough to stress about.

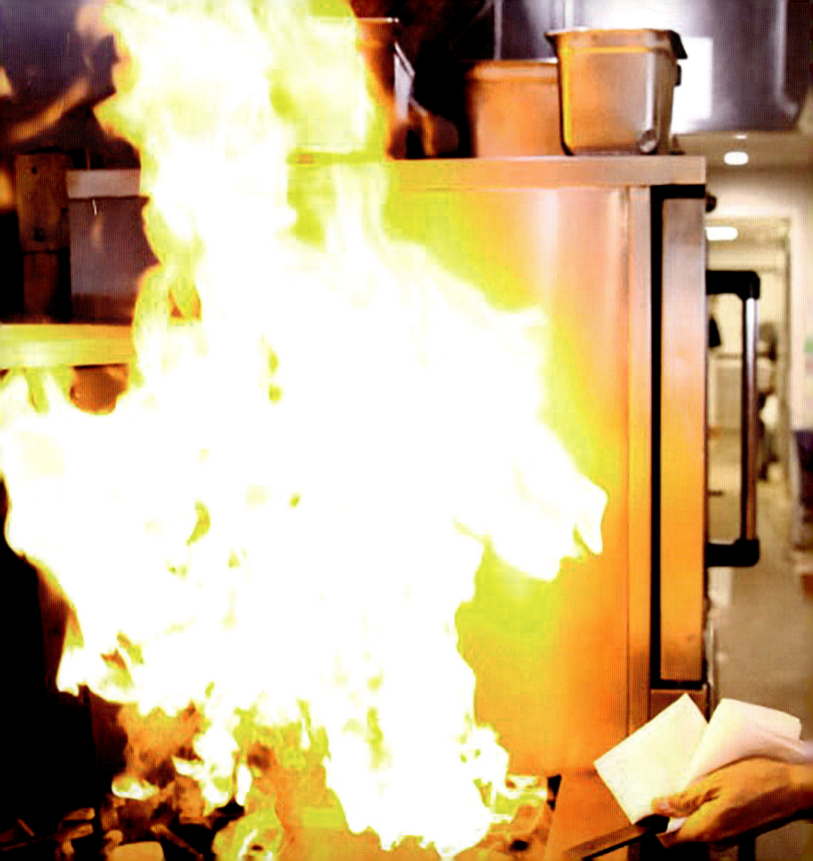

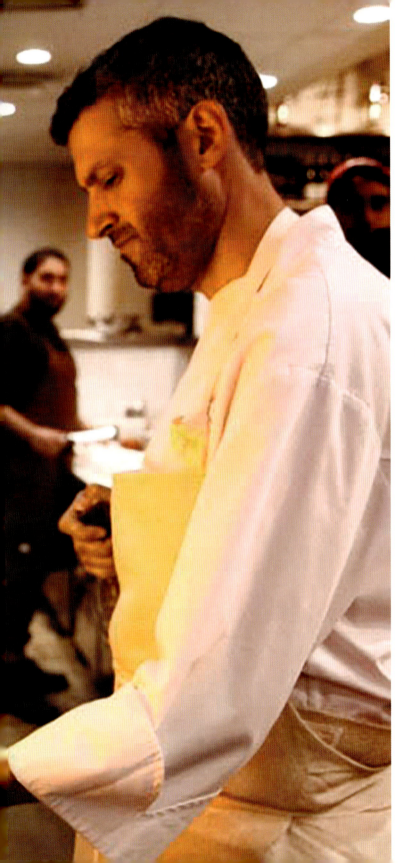

# 4
## Main
### Entrées + Entrée Salads

Our chefs not only create so-good-you-cannot-believe-they-are-healthy recipes, but they also hand over the reins and give you the tools to prepare these same crave-worthy dishes in your kitchen. We encourage you to make these meals your own. There are no rules. Just have fun!

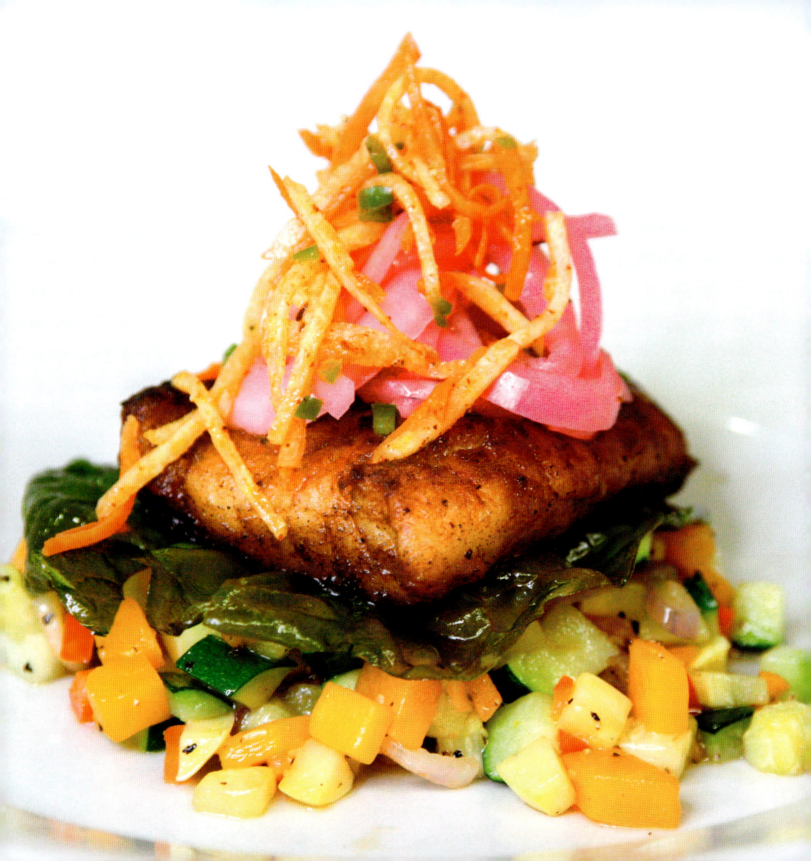

# Sweet Potato Snapper
## Café Vermilionville

**Makes 4 servings**

A virtual rainbow of colors towers over the plate, creating an off-the-charts wow factor.

- 4 snapper fillets, 5-6 ounces each
- ½ teaspoon sea salt
- ½ teaspoon freshly ground black pepper
- 2 tablespoons sweet potato flour
- 4 teaspoons light olive oil
- ½ cup Butternut Squash Hash (page 158)
- 4 large leaves Swiss chard, pan-fried until crispy
- ½ cup Jicama Slaw (page 95)
- ¼ cup Pickled Red Onions (page 163)

Preheat oven to 400 degrees. Lightly dust fish with salt, pepper, and flour. Heat oil in an oven-safe saucepan and sear fish on each side. Finish in the oven for 5 minutes, until fish is firm to the touch.

To serve, form 2 tablespoons Butternut Squash Hash in a tight circle in the center of each plate. Top with a flat "sheet" of pan-fried Swiss chard. Arrange the seared fish on top, add 2 tablespoons Jicama Slaw, and garnish with Pickled Red Onions.

PER SERVING: 350 calories, 18 grams fat, 2.5 grams saturated fat, 390 mg sodium, 13 grams carbohydrate (10 grams net carbs), 3 grams fiber, 4 grams sugar (0 added sugar), 34 grams protein

GF, Low Carb

## Tip

If you can't find sweet potato flour in your local market, it's easy to find online at a reasonable price.

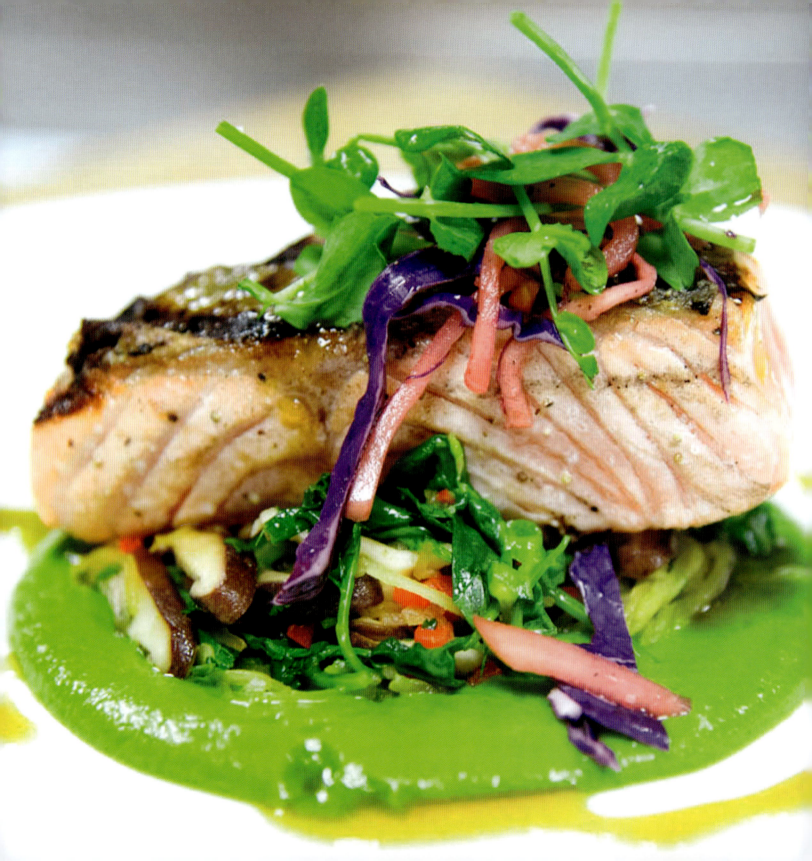

# Green Chili Glazed Grilled Salmon
## Commander's Palace

**Makes 4 servings**

Chef Carl Schaubhut created this dish during his stint at the Commander's Palace family of restaurants, and it's been a favorite ever since. Commander's Palace chefs de cuisine have served it up with a variety of different spins and twists, but this is the original version.

4 salmon fillets, 6 ounces each
¼ cup Green Chili Glaze (recipe follows)
1 cup Minted Pea Puree (recipe follows)
2 cups Sambal Vegetable Stir Fry (page 166)
1 cup Mirliton Salad (recipe follows)

Grill salmon fillets over medium-high heat for 2-3 minutes on each side for rare; 3-4 minutes on each side for medium. Spoon 1 tablespoon Green Chili Glaze over each fillet, and finish in oven at 300 degrees for 3 minutes until cooked to medium rare or 5 minutes until cooked to medium.

Spread 2 tablespoons warm Minted Pea Puree in a circle on bottom of each plate. Top with ½ cup Sambal Vegetable Stir Fry. Perch glazed salmon over the top of the stir fry. Top with ¼ cup Mirliton Salad. Drizzle Green Chili Glaze around the plate and serve.

**PER SERVING:** 440 calories, 24 grams fat, 5 grams saturated fat, 260 mg sodium, 18 grams carbohydrate (15 grams net carbs), 3 grams fiber, 8 grams sugar (3 grams added sugar), 38 grams protein

## GREEN CHILI GLAZE

### Makes approximately ¼ cup

- ½ tablespoon minced ginger
- ½ tablespoon minced garlic
- ½ tablespoon minced green onion
- ¼ cup light corn syrup
- ¼ cup rice wine vinegar
- ½ poblano chili, roasted, peeled, and seeded
- ½ small fresh jalapeño, roasted, peeled, and seeded
- ¼ orange, zested
- ½ lime, juiced
- 1 tablespoon reduced sodium soy sauce

In a saucepan over medium heat, sweat ginger, garlic, and green onion for 5 minutes. Add corn syrup and vinegar and reduce by half. Add remaining glaze ingredients and return to a simmer. Simmer 5 minutes, remove from heat, and allow to cool. Puree in blender then strain.

## MINTED PEA PUREE

### Makes approximately 1 cup

- 1 clove garlic, chopped
- ¼ onion, diced
- 1 cup fresh green peas (substitute fresh favas or fresh soybeans)
- 1 cup milk (reduced fat cow's milk or unsweetened coconut milk)
- 5 fresh mint leaves
- 5 fresh basil leaves
- ½ cup packed fresh spinach
- ½ lemon, zested and juiced
- ½ teaspoon sea salt
- ½ teaspoon freshly ground black pepper

In a small pot, sweat garlic and onion. Add peas and enough milk to barely cover. Bring to a boil then turn off the heat. Drain milk into a small bowl and reserve. Transfer cooked onion, garlic, and peas to a blender. Add mint, basil, spinach, lemon zest, and lemon juice to pea mixture. Season with salt and pepper. Blend slowly, adding reserved milk until mixture reaches a thick consistency. Gradually increase the speed of blender. Blend on high for 5 minutes. Strain through a mesh strainer for a silkier consistency.

## MIRLITON SALAD

### Makes approximately 1 cup

- ¼ cup Ginger Pickled Mirliton (page 163)
- ¼ cup shaped Napa cabbage
- ¼ cup shaved red cabbage
- ¼ cup shaved bok choy
- 1 green onion, diced
- ¼ cup chopped cilantro

Toss Ginger Pickled Mirliton with Napa cabbage, red cabbage, bok choy, green onion, and cilantro.

# Chef Meg Bickford
## Executive Chef, Commander's Palace

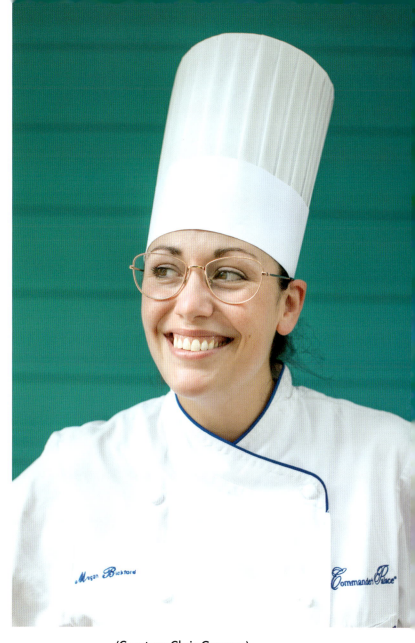

The first female executive chef in the 130-year history of Commander's Palace, Chef Meg leads with love, creativity, and compassion, while continuing to push culinary boundaries.

Growing up in New Orleans with family down the bayou, the kitchen has always been the center of Chef Meg's world. Summers growing up were spent fishing at her uncle's camp in South Louisiana; her downtime these days is centered on her daughter Stella and husband Richard—also a chef—often cooking with family and friends.

A brilliant and collaborative chef, she's also quite possibly the perfect Eat Fit chef-partner. Our team has a standing appointment in the kitchen with Chef Meg each month, where she catches us up on the latest menu, prepares the new dishes, and shares recipe details to confirm her hunch that they fit Eat Fit.

Meg leads by example in all that she does, and for that, we are grateful.

(Courtesy Chris Granger)

*"Food is such a powerful thing. It's the center of our celebrations, it nourishes our spirit and our soul. As I create new dishes for our menu, it's important to me to include Eat Fit cuisine that nourishes our body, as well."* —Chef Meg Bickford

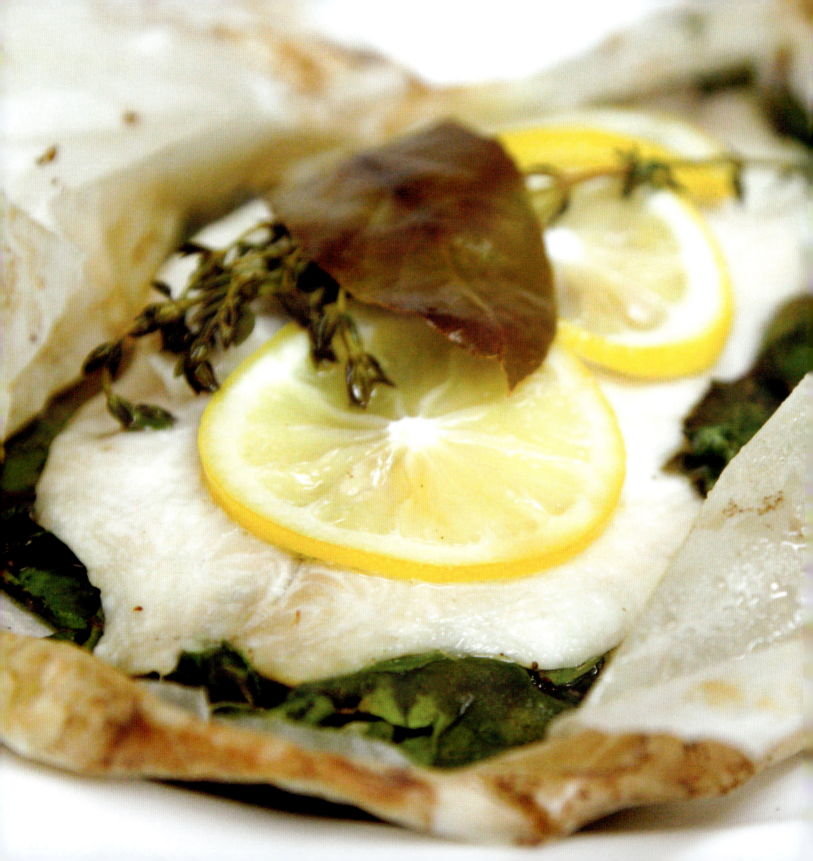

# Pompano en Papillote
## Blue Dog Café

**Makes 4 servings**

Loosely translated as "paper-wrapped fish," this recipe is simple, low carb, and protein rich. Best of all, nearly all of its ingredients can be found locally, no matter the season.

- 2 lemons, sliced ¼-inch thick
- 8 sprigs thyme
- 4 bay leaves
- 8 garlic cloves, thinly sliced
- ¼ cup cold-pressed pecan oil or extra virgin olive oil
- 4 pompano fillets, 7-9 ounces each, skin and bones removed
- ¼ teaspoon sea salt
- ¼ teaspoon freshly ground black pepper
- 1 cup fresh Swiss chard
- Fresh basil for garnish

Preheat oven to 400 degrees. Cut 4 pieces of parchment paper about 2 inches longer than the fish. Fold each paper in half lengthwise, then open it flat. Arrange lemon slices, thyme, bay leaves, and sliced garlic on one half of the paper. Drizzle oil on top of the herbs and use the rest to fully coat each fillet.

Season each side of fillets with salt and pepper. Place fillets on top of the lemon and herbs on each parchment paper, then add a handful of Swiss chard to each. Fold the other parchment half over the fish and roll the edges to seal the fish tightly. The "bags" should be formed in the shape of the fish. Place the bags onto the baking sheet and bake 10-12 minutes. When done, cut away the top of the bag and garnish with fresh chopped basil.

**PER SERVING:** 410 calories, 25 grams fat, 4.5 grams saturated fat, 270 mg sodium, 5 grams carbohydrate (4 grams net carbs), 1 gram fiber, <1 gram sugar (0 added sugar), 41 grams protein
GF, Low Carb

## Ingredient Improv

If you have difficulty finding pompano at your supermarket, substitute any type of white flaky fish.

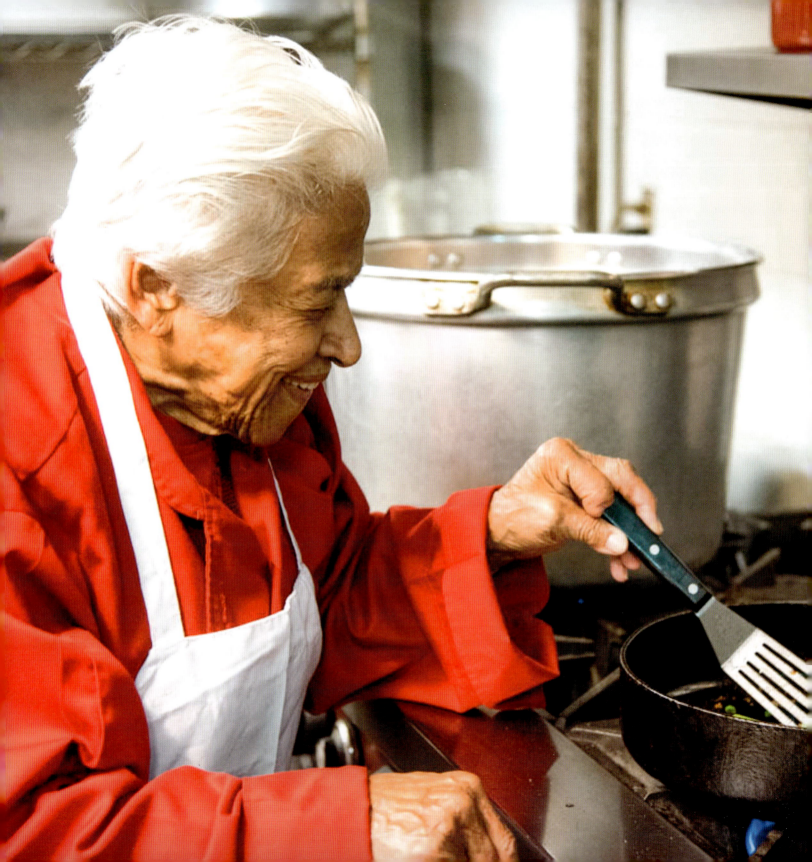

# Chef Leah Chase
## Dooky Chase's Restaurant

After experiencing a meal at Dooky Chase's, you'll have a sense of the two unexpected inspirations that Chef Leah Chase credited with influencing her view of life and the way she ran her restaurant.

One is Tupac Shakur:

> "Sometimes we lose people with great talent by not paying enough attention to them.
>
> I have a painting of Tupac Shakur, and people ask me, 'Why Tupac?' I once went to an art show and saw the most beautiful poem on the wall; it was written by Tupac. Why did we lose this brilliant man? Because he was a man that people didn't pay attention to and didn't give him the love he needed. He had two roads to take, he veered off of that right road, and he had nobody to help bring him back.
>
> I keep his picture to remind me to try to lift people up. Because you never know how you may help, what kind of impact you may have on their lives. And we often help ourselves, in the process."

The other inspiration is General George Patton. As she explains,

> "I have a print of General Patton on his horse, given to me by a friend. I admire that Patton set goals for himself and worked hard to achieve them. He would say, 'Lead me, follow me, or get the hell out of my way.' I can relate. I don't use that kind of language, but I can relate. You have in your mind what you want, what you want to accomplish, and just get it done."

When you have a meal at Dooky Chase's, you can feel both of these influences. Everyone is warm, welcoming, loving, listening, lifting us up. And in the back of the house, it's no nonsense and high expectations. Nothing less than perfect should leave the kitchen, and everyone plays a role in getting it done.

> **"People give me energy, I'm learning every day. No matter who you are, what you are, you can always learn."**
> —Chef Leah Chase

## Legacy /

Leah Chase passed away as this book was going to print. We are grateful that we had the opportunity to learn from this incredible woman who has been such a source of strength, unity, and inspiration for New Orleans and beyond.

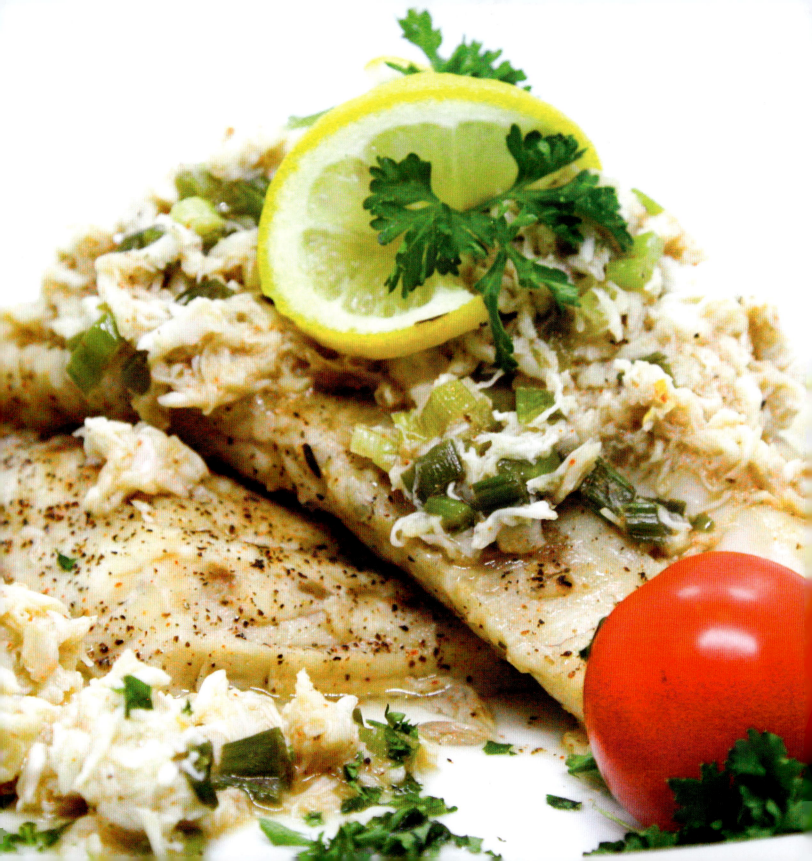

# Redfish Orleans
## Dooky Chase's Restaurant

**Makes 4 servings**

Family owned and operated since 1941, Dooky Chase's Restaurant boasts a clientele that includes U.S. presidents, Grammy Award-winning musicians, professional athletes, and world-renowned authors. Best known for its down-home Southern fare, the restaurant offers a full menu of New Orleans favorites such as red beans and rice, shrimp Creole, gumbo, and truly inspired seafood dishes like this one.

- 1 tablespoon unsalted butter
- 2 cups water
- 1 teaspoon cayenne pepper
- 1 teaspoon sea salt
- 4 redfish fillets, 7-9 ounces each
- 1 cup Orleans Sauce (recipe follows)
- 1 lemon, sliced into thin wheels
- 4 cherry tomatoes
- ¼ cup fresh parsley

In a deep skillet, bring butter and water to a boil. Add cayenne and salt. Reduce heat. Place fish in water and poach until fish is just cooked through, about 5-6 minutes. (Reserve 2 tablespoons liquid to make Orleans Sauce.) Once fish is cooked, transfer to a platter. To serve, top each fillet with ¼ cup of Orleans Sauce and garnish with lemon, tomato, and fresh parsley.

## ORLEANS SAUCE

**Makes approximately 1 cup**

- 1 tablespoon unsalted butter
- ½ tablespoon whole wheat pastry flour or brown rice flour
- ¼ cup evaporated milk
- 2 tablespoons liquid reserved from poaching redfish
- 2 tablespoons white wine
- ½ tablespoon Lea & Perrins Worcestershire sauce
- ½ teaspoon sea salt
- ½ teaspoon white pepper
- 1 cup lump crabmeat

In a medium pot, melt butter over medium heat. Add flour and stir well. Do not brown. Whisk in milk, reserved liquid, and wine until smooth. Add Worcestershire sauce, sea salt, and white pepper. Fold crabmeat into sauce and simmer for 3 minutes, or until crabmeat is heated through.

**PER SERVING:** 570 calories, 23 grams fat, 7 grams saturated fat, 530 mg sodium, 4 grams carbohydrate (4 grams net carbs), <1 gram fiber, 2 grams sugar (0 added sugar), 80 grams protein

LOW CARB

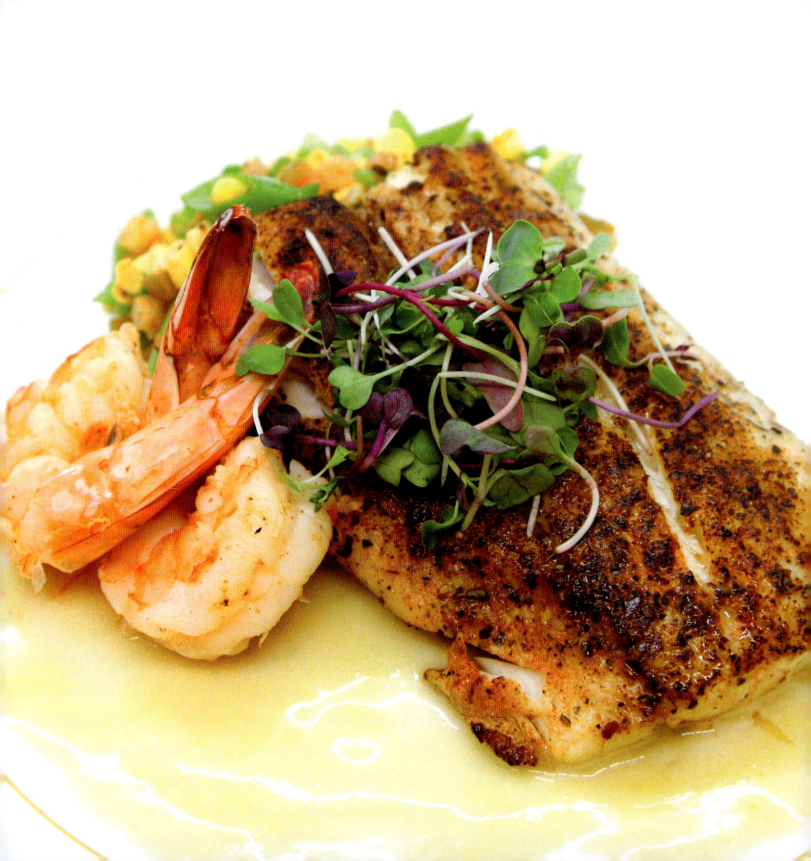

# Grilled Fish + Shrimp with Corn Maque Choux + Creole Lemon Vinaigrette

*Broussard's Restaurant*

**Makes 4 servings**

For more than a century, Broussard's has been delighting its customers with a menu that showcases a perfect marriage of Creole and French cuisines. Allowing you to play celebrity chef in your own kitchen, this recipe is quintessentially New Orleans, but don't be afraid to put your own signature on it! Any type of fresh fish will perform well here.

- 4 fresh fish fillets, 7-9 ounces each
- 8 jumbo shrimp, peeled and deveined
- 4 tablespoons olive oil, divided
- ½ teaspoon sea salt, divided
- ½ teaspoon freshly ground black pepper, divided
- 4 stalks of corn, cleaned and cut off the cob
- 1 cup diced red bell peppers
- 4 tablespoons diced red onion
- 4 tablespoons sliced green onion
- ¼ teaspoon cayenne pepper
- ½ cup Creole Lemon Vinaigrette (page 176)

Coat fish and shrimp with 2 tablespoons olive oil and season with a pinch each of salt and pepper. Grill over medium-high heat.

Heat remaining 2 tablespoons olive oil in a skillet over medium heat. Add corn, red peppers, and red onion and sauté until tender. Remove corn mixture from stove, fold in green onion, and season with cayenne and remaining salt and pepper.

Place corn mixture in the center of a serving plate, top with fish and shrimp, and drizzle with Creole Lemon Vinaigrette.

**PER SERVING:** 620 calories, 33 grams fat, 6 grams saturated fat, 450 mg sodium, 25 grams carbohydrate (22 grams net carbs), 3 grams fiber, 11 grams sugar (2 grams added sugar), 61 grams protein
**GF**

## Nutrition Bite

If you're watching carbs, use diced yellow pepper in place of corn.

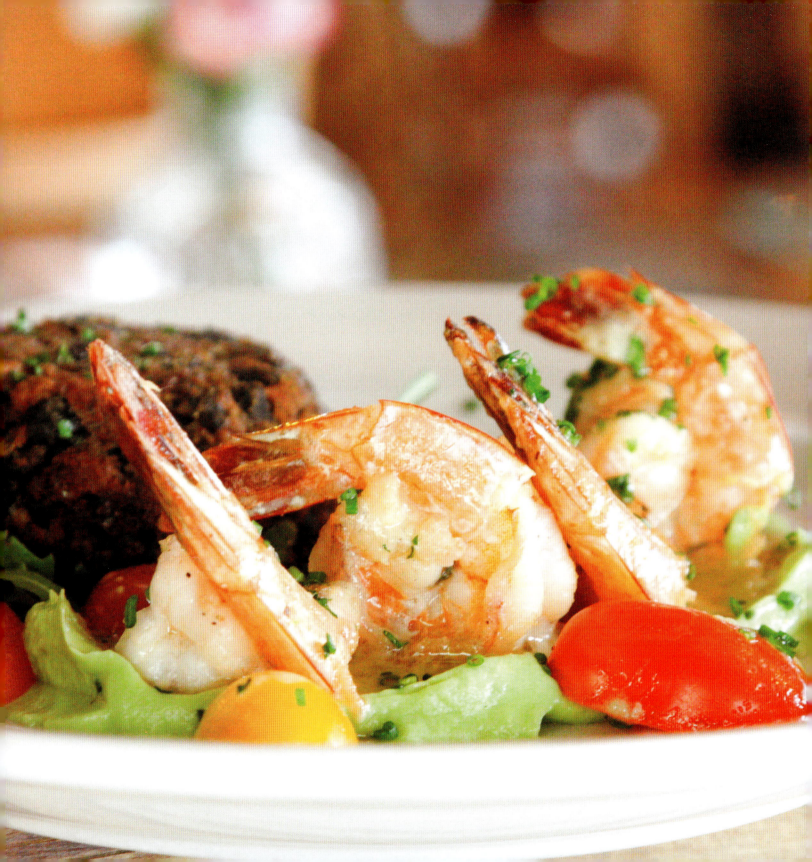

# Grilled Shrimp with Black Bean Cake + Avocado Puree
## Café Degas

**Makes 8 servings**

The creative presentation of this dish by Café Degas elevates everyday ingredients to a whole new level of culinary expression.

### For the Black Bean Cake

6 tablespoons extra virgin olive oil, divided
1 small onion, diced
½ teaspoon ground cumin
½ teaspoon ground coriander
½ teaspoon sea salt
½ teaspoon freshly ground black pepper
2 teaspoons minced garlic
28 ounces canned black beans, drained and rinsed
2 tablespoons chopped fresh cilantro
1 egg, lightly beaten
1 lime, juiced
2 teaspoons hot sauce
4-8 tablespoons whole wheat pastry flour

### For the Shrimp

1 tablespoon light olive oil
1 tablespoon butter, divided
1 pound 16/20 count shrimp, peeled with tail on
1 teaspoon minced garlic
1 teaspoon chopped fresh chives
1 teaspoon chopped fresh parsley
½ tablespoon lemon juice
1 cup halved cherry tomatoes, for garnish
1 cup Avocado Puree, for garnish (recipe follows)

**Prepare the Black Bean Cake:** Heat 2 tablespoons oil in a medium sauté pan over medium heat. Add onion, cumin, coriander, salt, and pepper and cook until the onion is soft and lightly caramelized, about 3 minutes. Add garlic and cook until fragrant, about 30 seconds. Remove pan from heat and set aside to cool.

In a medium mixing bowl, mash black beans until relatively smooth, with no whole beans remaining. Stir in the cooled onion mixture, cilantro, beaten egg, lime juice, and hot sauce. Mix well. Add 2 tablespoons of whole wheat flour and mix well. Gradually mix in additional flour 1 tablespoon at a time, as needed, until the mixture binds.

Heat remaining oil in a large non-stick pan over medium heat. Use ½ cup measure to make 8 patties. Gently sear the cakes until browned on both sides and heated through, about 2 minutes per side. Place black bean cakes into oven on low heat to keep warm until ready to serve.

**Sauté the Shrimp:** In a large pan over high heat, heat 1 tablespoon oil and ½ tablespoon butter. Sear shrimp in olive oil and butter for about 2 minutes. Turn shrimp and add garlic, chives, and parsley. Cook for 1 minute or until garlic is slightly browned, then stir in lemon juice and heat for another minute. Remove from heat and add remaining ½ tablespoon butter.

Plate each bean cake. Arrange the shrimp around the bean cake. Garnish with cherry tomatoes and a generous dollop of Avocado Puree. Drizzle with butter and juices from the pan and serve.

### AVOCADO PUREE

**Makes approximately 1 cup**

1 avocado, peeled, pitted, and mashed
¼ cup 2% plain Greek yogurt
2 tablespoons lemon juice
½ clove fresh garlic, minced
1 pinch sea salt
1 pinch freshly ground black pepper

In a blender, puree avocado, Greek yogurt, lemon juice, garlic, salt, pepper, and 1 tablespoon water until smooth and creamy. If needed, add more water 1 tablespoon at a time, until puree reaches a whipped, mousse-like consistency.

PER SERVING: 410 calories, 20 grams fat, 4.5 grams saturated fat, 190 mg sodium, 35 grams carbohydrate (23 grams net carbs), 12 grams fiber, 2 grams sugar (0 added sugar), 24 grams protein

Molly and Eat Fit Acadiana's Yvette Quantz enjoying Sweet Potato Snapper (page 99)

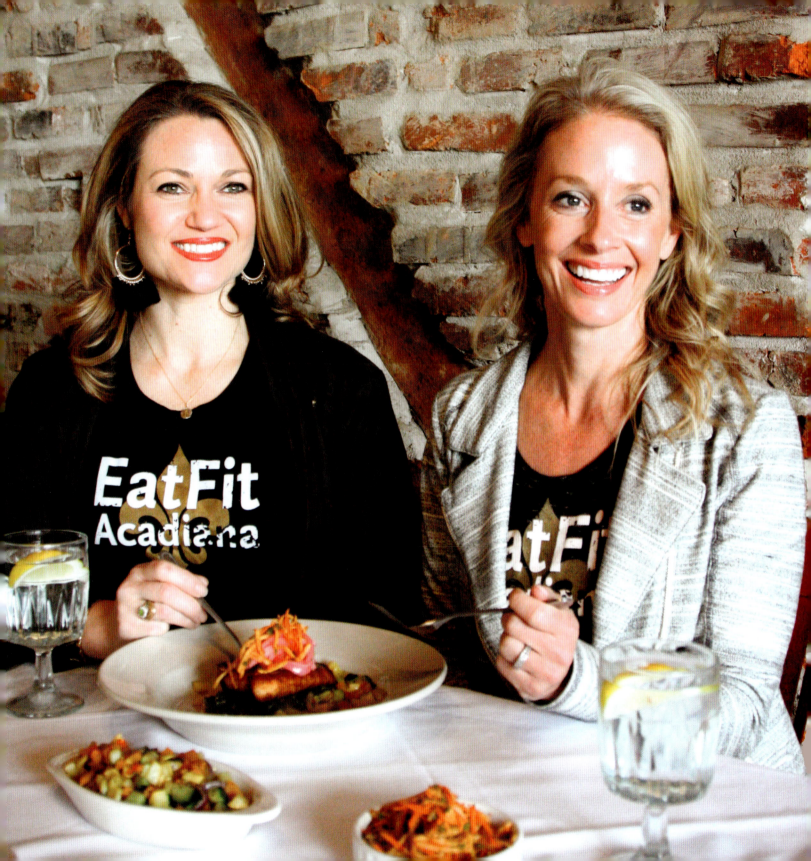

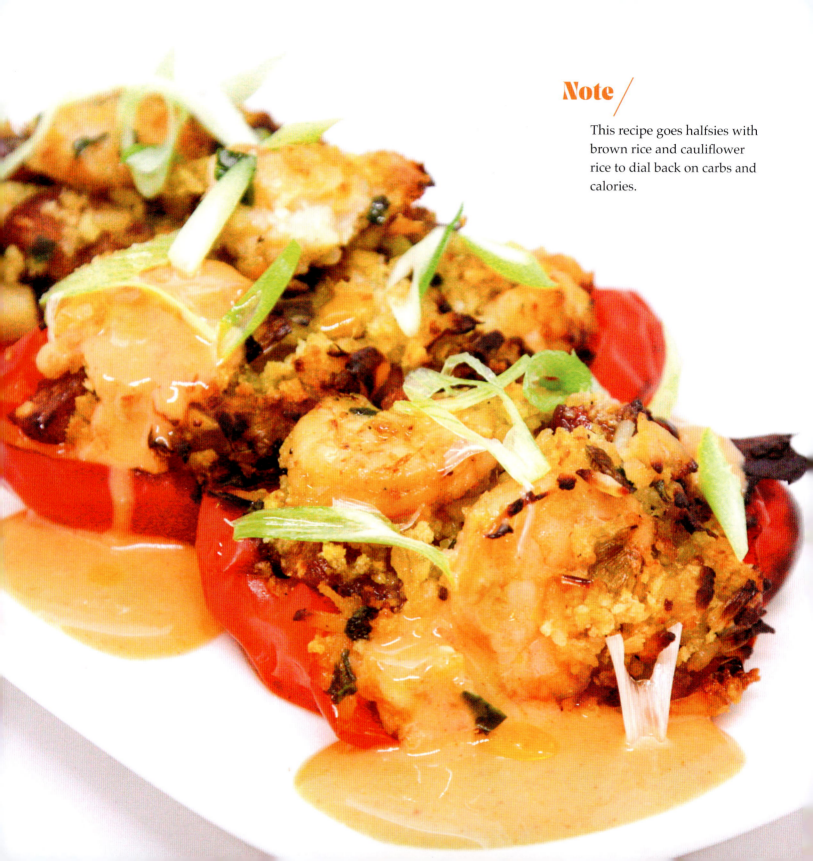

## Note

This recipe goes halfsies with brown rice and cauliflower rice to dial back on carbs and calories.

# Shrimp + Mirliton Stuffed Peppers
## Chef Carl Schaubhut

**Makes 8 servings**

In the South, bell peppers are typically stuffed with ground beef and white rice. But we much prefer Chef Carl's smoky stuffed peppers, a clever and artistic version of this traditional Southern delight.

- ¼ cup light olive oil
- 1 pound turkey tasso, small diced
- 4 cloves garlic, minced
- 1 fresh jalapeño, minced
- 2 red bell peppers, diced
- 2 mirlitons, medium diced
- 1 yellow onion, diced
- 3 ribs celery, diced
- ¼ teaspoon sea salt
- 1 teaspoon ground black pepper
- 1 teaspoon cayenne pepper
- 1 teaspoon dried oregano
- 1 teaspoon dried basil
- 1 teaspoon dried thyme
- 1 teaspoon granulated garlic
- 1 teaspoon granulated onion
- 1 cup uncooked brown rice
- ¼ cup white wine
- 2 cups unsalted seafood or chicken stock
- 1 pound medium Gulf shrimp, peeled
- ¼ cup Steen's cane vinegar
- ¼ cup Lea & Perrins Worcestershire sauce
- 2 tablespoons hot sauce
- ½ cup chopped fresh parsley
- 1 cup julienned green onions
- 2 cups riced cauliflower
- 8 red bell peppers, halved and seeded
- 1 tablespoon butter
- ½ cup grated Parmesan cheese
- ½ cup Chipotle Crema (page 184)

Preheat oven to 400 degrees. Add oil to a large pot over medium heat. Once oil is shimmering, add tasso and cook until brown, then remove from heat.

In a sauté pan, add garlic and jalapeño and cook until brown. Mix in diced red peppers, mirlitons, onion, celery, salt, pepper, and cayenne then cook for 10 minutes. Season with oregano, basil, thyme, granulated garlic, and granulated onion then cook for 5 more minutes. Add rice and sauté for 5 minutes.

Add wine to deglaze pan. Pour in stock then bring to a boil, stirring continuously. Reduce heat and simmer covered for 30 minutes or until rice is cooked. Mix in tasso, shrimp, vinegar, Worcestershire, hot sauce, parsley, green onions, and riced cauliflower. Remove from heat, spread on sheet pan, and let cool.

Fill each halved pepper with the rice stuffing. Place a dot of butter on top of each pepper half and sprinkle with Parmesan cheese. Bake until pepper is tender, about 30-35 minutes. Serve drizzled with Chipotle Crema.

**PER SERVING:** 340 calories, 13 grams fat, 3.5 grams saturated fat, 820 mg sodium, 29 grams carbohydrate (21 grams net carbs), 8 grams fiber, 13 grams sugar (0 added sugar), 25 grams protein

## Tip /
Look for Savoie's turkey tasso in local stores.

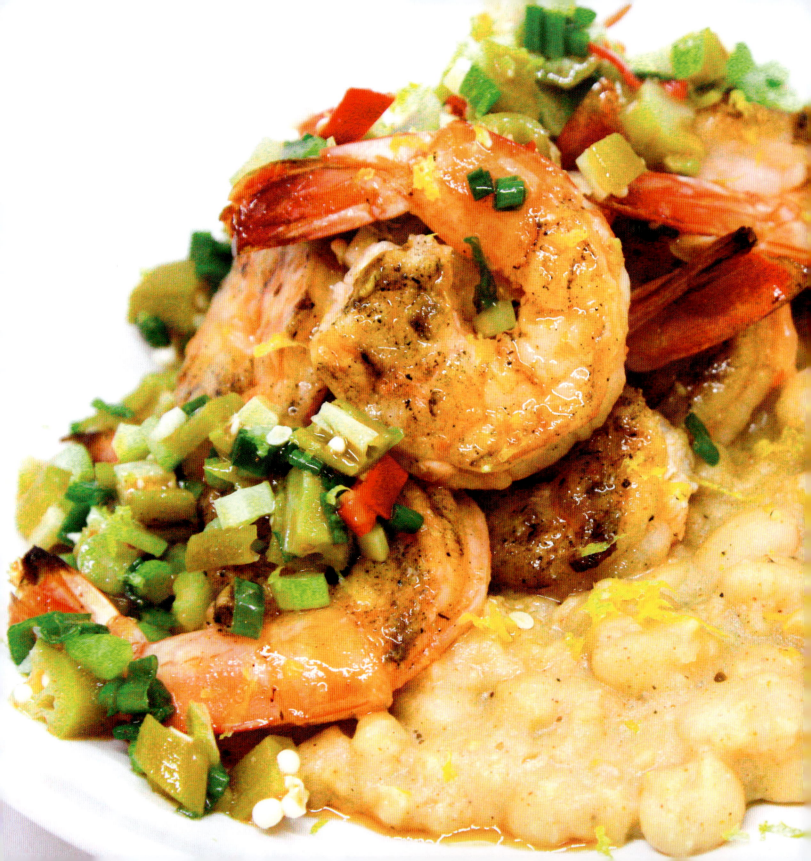

# Grilled Garlic Shrimp with White Beans + Pickled Okra Giardiniera

## Chef Carl Schaubhut

**Makes 8 Servings**

This entrée is no less than a divine south Louisiana comfort food. Chef Carl creates a beautiful Eat Fit dish that warms our souls while nourishing our bodies.

- 2 pounds large shrimp, peeled
- 1 tablespoon minced garlic
- 1 tablespoon low-sodium Creole seasoning
- 1 tablespoon light olive oil
- ¼ cup white wine
- 1 teaspoon chopped fresh thyme
- 1 lemon, juiced
- 4 cups White Beans (page 161)
- ½ cup Pickled Okra Giardiniera (recipe follows)
- 1 tablespoon extra virgin olive oil

In a mixing bowl, toss shrimp with garlic and Creole seasoning.

Heat a large skillet over medium-high heat. Add oil to pan, then add the seasoned shrimp, taking care not to overcrowd the pan. Cook shrimp about 3 minutes, flip, and cook another 2 minutes, until lightly browned. Add white wine to deglaze. Cook 30 seconds to reduce, then add thyme and lemon juice. Remove from heat. Place shrimp over ½ cup of White Beans, top with 1 tablespoon Pickled Okra Giardiniera, finish with a drizzle of extra virgin olive oil, and serve.

### PICKLED OKRA GIARDINIERA

**Makes approximately 2½ cups**

- 8 ounces jarred pickled okra, drained and diced
- ½ red onion, diced
- 8 ounces jarred pickled pepperoncini peppers, drained and sliced
- 1½ teaspoons minced garlic
- ½ cup chopped fresh parsley
- 1 rib celery, diced
- 1 tablespoon extra virgin olive oil
- 2 tablespoons red wine vinegar
- ½ teaspoon red chili pepper flakes
- ½ lemon, zested

Combine all ingredients and mix well. Refrigerate for at least 4 hours. May be prepared a day in advance.

**PER SERVING:** 240 calories, 5 grams fat, 0.5 gram saturated fat, 480 mg sodium, 21 grams carbohydrate (15 grams net carbs), 6 grams fiber, 3 grams sugar (0 added sugar), 28 grams protein

## Love It Later

We personally love to eat the leftover Pickled Okra by the spoonful straight out of the jar. It's also delish on salads, sandwiches, or as part of a big cheese board for guests.

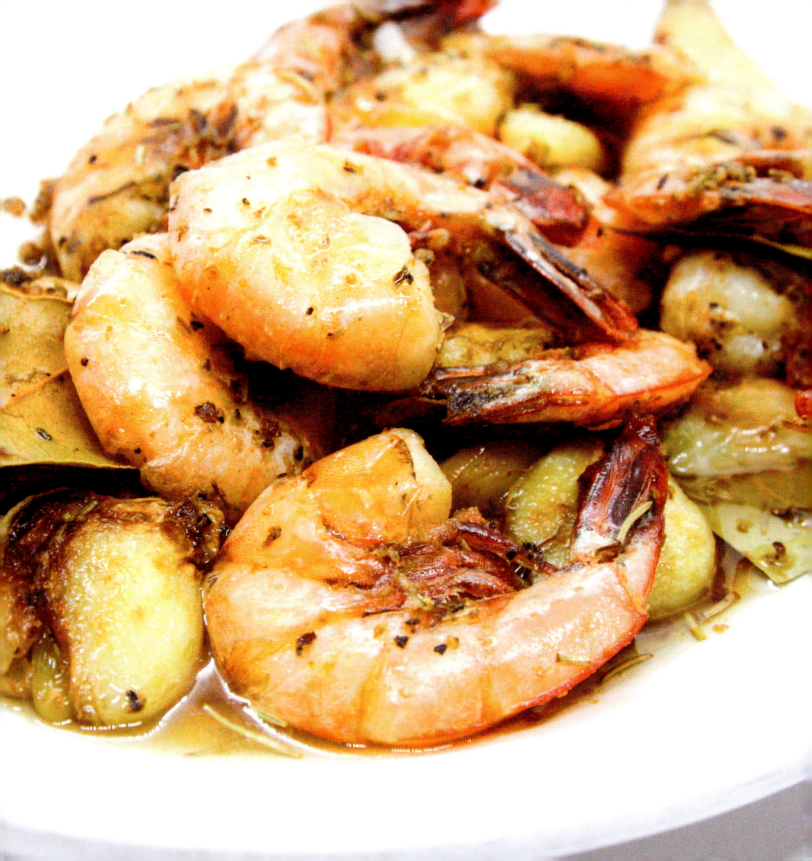

# Shrimp Mosca
## Mosca's Restaurant

**Makes 6 servings**

For decades, Mosca's loyal patrons have enjoyed a dining experience deeply rooted in Italian tradition and a family-friendly atmosphere. Served on a platter for sharing, Shrimp Mosca is centered on pure, simple, and clean ingredients.

1½ pounds 16/20 count jumbo shrimp, shells on
⅓ cup light olive oil
1 teaspoon sea salt
10 garlic cloves, crushed
3 bay leaves
1 teaspoon dried rosemary
1 teaspoon dried oregano
1 teaspoon freshly ground black pepper
¼ cup white wine
1 lemon, cut into wedges (optional)

Combine shrimp, olive oil, salt, garlic, bay leaves, rosemary, oregano, and pepper in a large skillet. Cook over medium-high heat, stirring occasionally for 10 minutes or just until shrimp have turned that pretty, orange color and the liquid produced by shrimp has almost completely evaporated.

Remove from heat and add wine. Return pan to heat, reduce to low, and cook at a low simmer until the liquid is reduced by half, about 5-7 minutes. Add a squeeze of lemon (Mosca's doesn't serve it with lemon, but a lot of people like to add it) and serve immediately.

**PER SERVING:** 220 calories, 13 grams fat, 2 grams saturated fat, 360 mg sodium, 3 grams carbohydrate (3 grams net carbs), 0 fiber, 0 sugar, 23 grams protein
**GF, Low Carb**

## Tip

If shrimp are frozen, soak them in water for 30 minutes before cooking. This helps to loosen the shell when peeling.

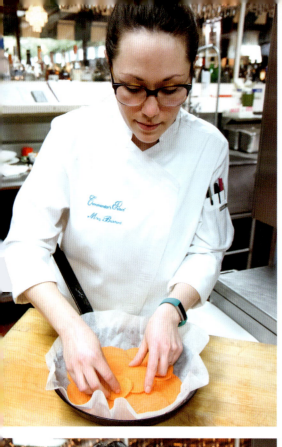
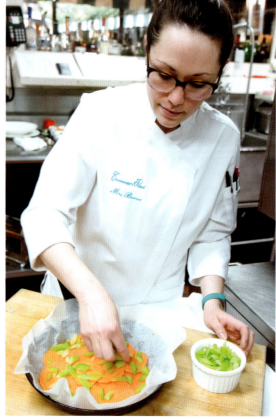
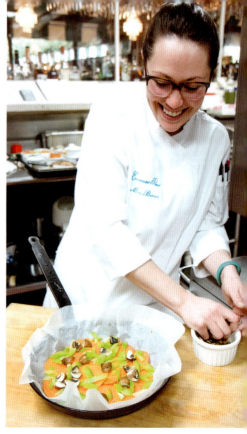
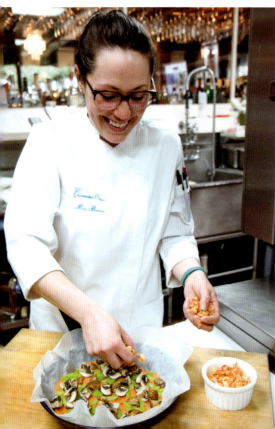
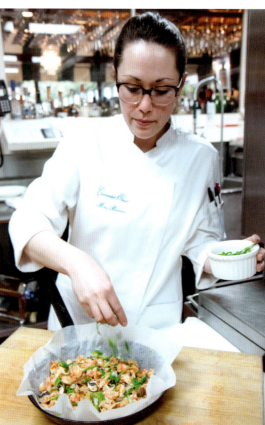
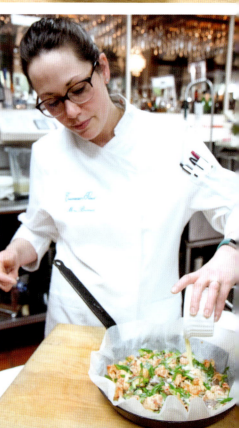

# Crawfish Boil Quiche
## Commander's Palace

**Makes 6 servings**

This make-ahead dish is a great way to repurpose leftover crawfish from last weekend's boil. Bursting with flavor, Commander's Palace Crawfish Boil Quiche will get you invited back to the party again and again.

1 sweet potato, baked to a soft yet firm texture, thinly sliced
½ cup mushrooms, boiled, thinly sliced
½ cup boiled, peeled crawfish tails
½ cup steamed green onions, julienned
½ cup steamed celery, julienned
6 eggs
1 cup milk (reduced fat cow's milk or unsweetened coconut milk)

Preheat oven to 350 degrees. Spray a 9-inch cast-iron pan with nonstick cooking spray and line with wax paper, leaving plenty of extra paper around the rim. Push the waxed paper into the sides and bottom of the pan so it starts to stick and takes the shape of the pan.

Layer the sliced potatoes in a circular pattern, overlapping slightly to form the bottom crust. Smash the potatoes down into the bottom of the pan to seal the crust into place. As if you were making a pizza, layer the mushrooms, crawfish, and steamed vegetables. Heat in the oven for 15 minutes, or until the mixture is hot all the way through.

Meanwhile, in a blender, combine eggs and milk and blend 20 seconds until fluffy. Let the eggs sit, then blend for an additional 30 seconds to incorporate as much air as possible to make them light and fluffy. Pour eggs evenly over the top of the vegetables and return to the oven until the quiche is just set, about 10-13 minutes. Remove from the oven and allow to sit for 5 minutes.

To serve, hold the extra waxed paper on each side of the cast-iron skillet and remove the quiche to a cutting board. Cut with a pizza wheel or sharp knife and serve.

**PER SERVING:** 130 calories, 6 grams fat, 2 grams saturated fat, 125 mg sodium, 8 grams carbohydrate (7 grams net carbs), 1 gram fiber, 2 grams sugar (0 added sugar), 11 grams protein
GF, Low Carb, Low Sodium

Meg Bickford, executive chef at Commander's Palace.

## Tip

Not crawfish season? This recipe is easy enough to make on a weekday without boiling 30 pounds of crawfish. Just boil a small batch on the stovetop with a dash of seafood seasoning boil.

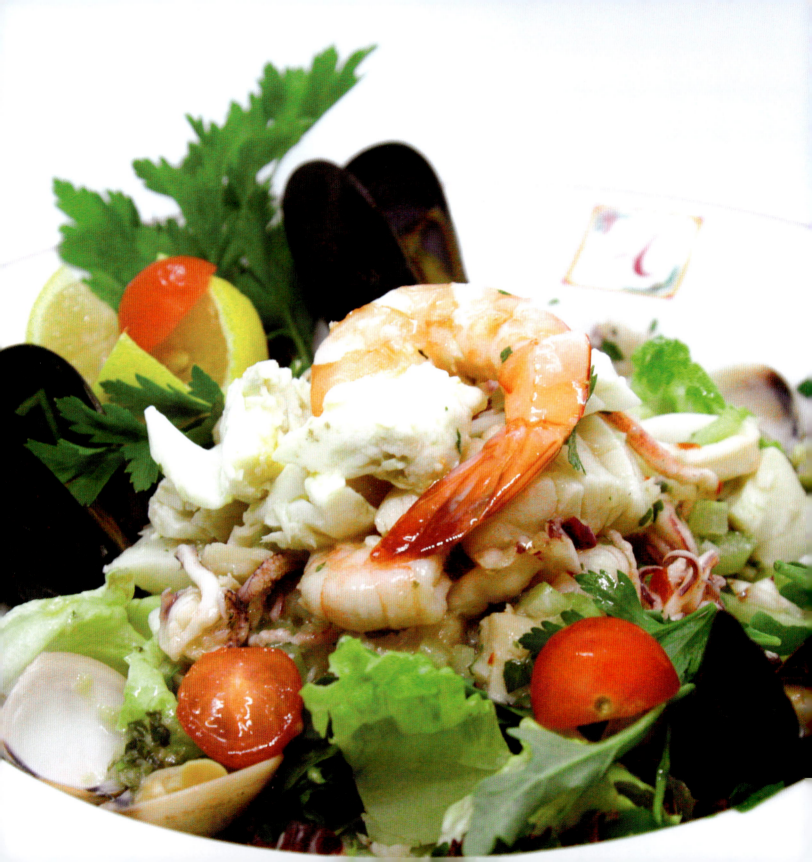

# Frutti di Mare Portofino
## Andrea's Restaurant

**Makes 6 servings**

Have a favorite seafood you would like to include in this recipe? No problem. This chilled dish flourishes with *any* fresh seafood. Think salmon, crawfish, or even octopus. You simply can't go wrong.

**For the Poached Seafood**
- ½ tablespoon vinegar
- 1 bay leaf
- ¼ pound scallops
- ½ pound squid, cleaned
- ½ pound shrimp, peeled and deveined
- ½ pound red snapper fillets

**For the Sautéed Seafood**
- 2 tablespoons extra virgin olive oil
- 1 teaspoon chopped onion
- ½ teaspoon chopped garlic
- ⅛ teaspoon crushed red pepper flakes
- ⅛ teaspoon white pepper
- ¾ pound mussels, in shells
- ¼ cup dry white wine, such as Chardonnay
- ¾ pound clams, in shells

**For the Sauce**
- ½ cup extra virgin olive oil
- 2 tablespoons lemon juice
- ¼ cup dry white wine
- ½ teaspoon Lea & Perrins Worcestershire sauce
- 2 tablespoons chopped parsley
- 1 teaspoon chopped onion
- ¼ pound lump crabmeat, chilled
- 1 head Romaine lettuce, chopped

**Poach the Seafood:** Rinse all seafood. In a large pot, bring 4 quarts water, vinegar, and bay leaf to a boil. With a slotted spoon, carefully add scallops to the water and poach for 5 minutes, or until water returns to a boil. Remove and repeat with squid, shrimp, and snapper. Drain and refrigerate poached seafood.

**Sauté the Seafood:** Heat olive oil in a large skillet until hot. Sauté onion and garlic until translucent. Stir in red pepper flakes and white pepper. Place mussels in pan and add wine. Bring wine to a boil, reduce heat, and cover. Steam until mussels open, about 5 minutes. Remove mussels and set aside. Add clams to the skillet, cover, and steam until clams open. Transfer mussels and clams to a large bowl and refrigerate until cold. Remove half of the chilled clams and mussels from shells and chop coarsely.

Whisk together the sauce ingredients in a large bowl. Add chilled poached seafood, chopped mussels and clams, and lump crabmeat to the sauce and toss lightly. Serve atop lettuce and surrounded by mussels and clams in the shells.

**PER SERVING:** 470 calories, 27 grams fat, 4 grams saturated fat, 750 mg sodium, 11 grams carbohydrate (9 grams net carbs), 2 grams fiber, 2 grams sugar (0 added sugar), 43 grams protein

GF, Low Carb

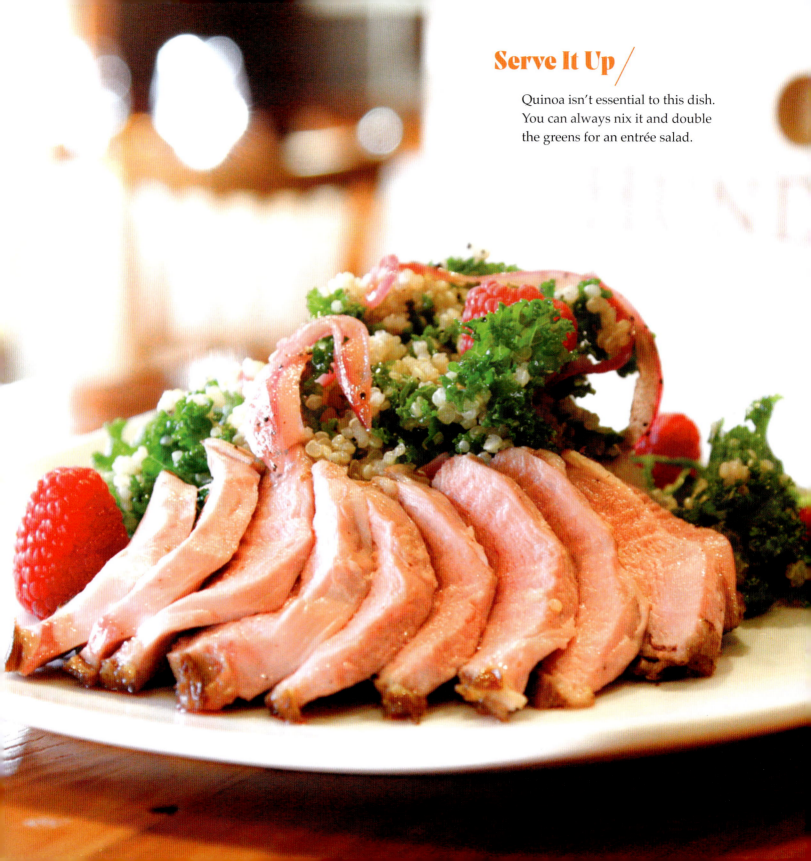

### Serve It Up /

Quinoa isn't essential to this dish. You can always nix it and double the greens for an entrée salad.

# Coffee Cured Duck Breast Salad with Quinoa + Kale
*Dakota Restaurant*

**Makes 6 servings**

Steen's cane syrup and coffee (use your favorite brew!) are the secret ingredients behind this recipe's sweet and savory bite. Don't get us wrong though. The duck, quinoa, kale, and raspberries play a big role in making this interesting recipe a hit with everyone who tries it.

**For the Duck**
- 2 quarts coffee
- 2 tablespoons sea salt
- 1 tablespoon freshly ground black pepper
- ½ cup Steen's cane syrup
- 6 duck breasts, 6 ounces each

**For the Salad**
- 3 cups cooked quinoa
- 6 cups kale, chopped
- ½ cup Poppyseed Berry Vinaigrette (page 177)
- ½ cup fresh raspberries for garnish
- ¼ shaved red onions for garnish

**Prepare the Duck in advance:** In a saucepan, heat coffee over medium heat. Bring to a simmer and stir in salt, pepper, and cane syrup until dissolved. Remove mixture from heat and allow to cool. Place mixture and duck breast in a covered container and refrigerate to brine for 12 hours or overnight.

Remove duck from brine, rinse, and pat dry. Sear duck breast in skillet over medium-high heat, skin side down, for 5 minutes on each side until medium to medium-rare. Cook a few minutes longer if you prefer your duck more well done. Let rest for 5 minutes before removing skin and slicing.

**Assemble the Salad:** In a mixing bowl, combine quinoa, kale, and Berry Poppyseed Vinaigrette. Toss until evenly coated. Pile into center of serving plates and top with sliced duck breast. Garnish with fresh raspberries and shaved red onions.

**PER SERVING:** 440 calories, 22 grams fat, 6 grams saturated fat, 140 mg sodium, 26 grams carbohydrate (22 grams net carbs), 4 grams fiber, 2 grams sugar (<1 gram added sugar), 36 grams protein
GF, Low Sodium

## Cost Saver
Skinless chicken thighs can be used in place of duck breasts.

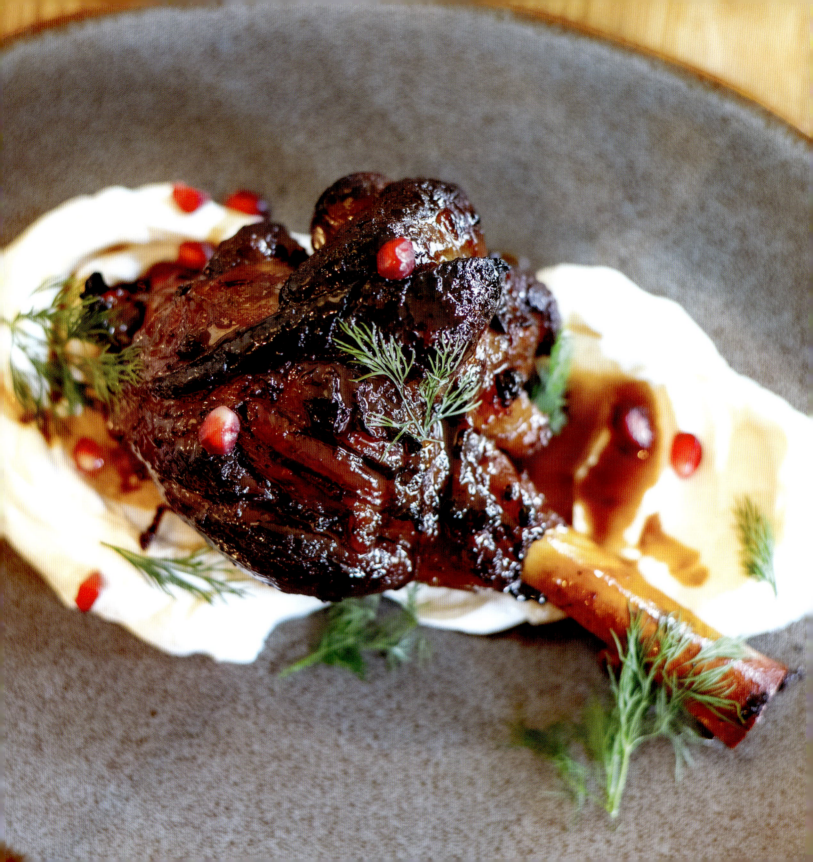

# Braised Lamb Shank with Pomegranate Glaze and Labneh
## *Saba*

**Makes 4 shanks for 4-8 servings**

A signature dish of Alon Shaya's for nearly a decade, elevating two symbolic foods—lamb and pomegranate—in a way that elicits a bit of surprise and also comfort. The tart sweetness of the pomegranate glaze perfectly complements the tender, fall-off-the-bone lamb; the bold flavors rounded out with creamy labneh.

4 lamb hind shanks, approximately 2-3 pounds each
8 cups cold water, divided
1½ tablespoons kosher salt
1 tablespoon dark brown sugar
¼ cup fresh-squeezed orange juice
3 fresh bay leaves
½ teaspoon whole black peppercorns
½ teaspoon whole allspice
4 sprigs fresh rosemary
1 cup ice
½ cup pomegranate molasses
¾ cup honey
3 tablespoons granulated sugar
3 cups pomegranate juice
1 cup Labneh (page 174)
1 teaspoon fresh dill
1 tablespoon fresh pomegranate seeds

Place lamb shanks in a container and allow to come to room temperature.

In a small pot over low heat, add 1 cup of water with 1½ tablespoons salt, along with brown sugar, orange juice, bay leaves, black peppercorns, allspice, and rosemary. Bring to a simmer for 2 minutes, until salt and sugar completely dissolve, creating a brine for the lamb.

While simmering, place 1 cup of ice and 2 cups of water in a large container that will fit lamb shanks and brine. Add the hot brine, including aromatics. Liquid should be warm to the touch, but not hot.

Add lamb shanks to liquid, cover, and refrigerate for 48 hours.

Five hours prior to serving the lamb shanks, preheat oven to 500 degrees. Remove lamb shanks and discard brine. Place lamb shanks on a baking sheet with a wire rack and roast until golden brown, about 15-20 minutes. Remove lamb shanks from oven and reduce temperature to 275 degrees.

Select a roasting pan that will fit the four lamb shanks with room for remaining ingredients. Place roasting pan on stovetop over low heat and add the remaining 5 cups of water along with the pomegranate molasses, honey, granulated sugar, and pomegranate juice. Stir until

## Pomegranate Molasses

Look for it on the international aisle in most grocery stores; it's also readily available at Middle Eastern specialty stores.

sugar has dissolved, about 2-3 minutes. Add roasted lamb shanks to pan and cover with foil or a tight-fitting lid.

Place pan in oven for about 2½ to 3 hours, until meat easily pulls from the bone. Once tender, remove pan from oven and carefully remove lamb shanks, ensuring meat does not fall off the bone.

For the pomegranate glaze, place roasting pan back on stovetop over high heat and reduce the braising liquid for about 10-15 minutes, or until sauce coats the back of a spoon.

Coat each lamb shank with a tablespoon of pomegranate glaze. To serve, smear a quarter cup or so of Labneh onto each plate. Top with lamb shank and garnish with fresh dill and pomegranate seeds.

PER SERVING: 370 calories, 15 grams fat, 7 grams saturated fat, 400 mg sodium, 5 grams carbohydrate (5 grams net carbs), 0 fiber, 3 grams sugar (1 gram added sugar), 49 grams protein
GF, Low Carb

## Lamb Alternative /

If you can't find lamb shank (or it's a bit pricey) Chef Alon recommends oxtail, turkey necks, or pork shank.

## Plan Ahead /

The hands-on time for this dish is relatively minimal, but do note the 48-hour marinade for the lamb—be sure to plan accordingly.

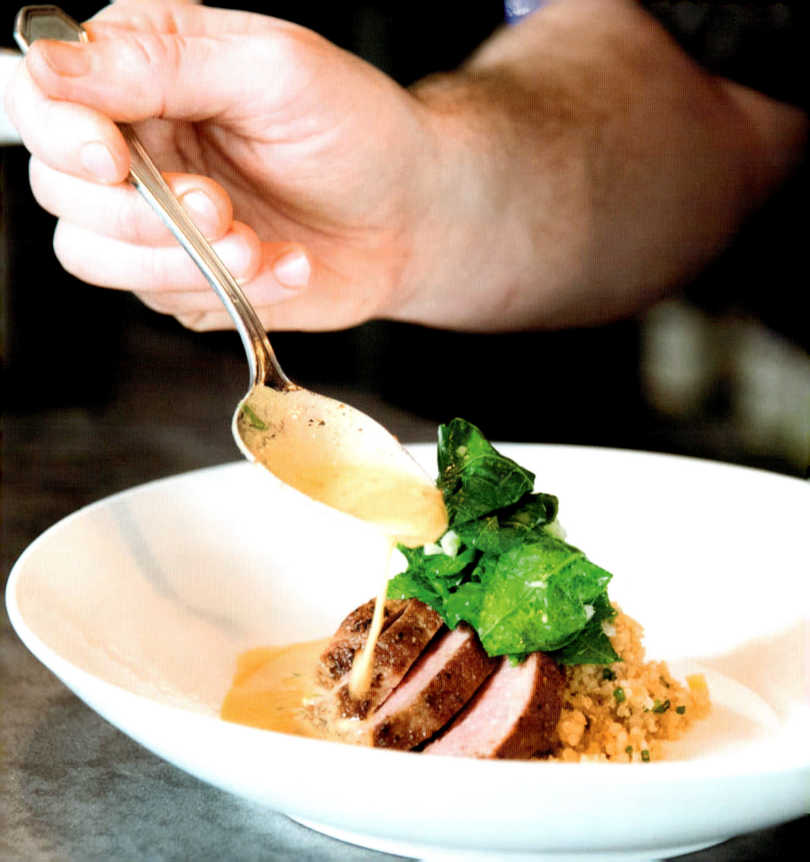

# Harissa Spiced Lamb Loin in Coconut Milk Curry + Quinoa

## Maypop

**Makes 6 servings**

I ordered this dish at Maypop, and I have been smitten with it ever since.

½ cup Harissa Paste (recipe follows)
¼ cup light olive oil
1½ pounds lamb loin, cleaned and trimmed
Dash of sea salt
¼ cup extra virgin olive oil
3 cups Quinoa (recipe follows)
12 leaves kale, collards or mustard greens, rinsed, destemmed, and roughly chopped
1½ cups warm Coconut Milk Curry (recipe follows)
Fresh herbs like basil or cilantro for garnish

Preheat oven to 350 degrees. Mix Harissa Paste and light olive oil and rub evenly over the surface of the lamb loin. Sprinkle with sea salt. Place lamb loin into a hot cast-iron pan, then place the pan directly into oven for 8 minutes or until lamb loin reads at least 110 degrees on an internal thermometer. Remove from oven and transfer to a cutting board. Allow lamb to rest for 10 minutes before slicing.

In a large sauté pan, heat extra virgin olive oil until it shimmers but doesn't smoke. Add the greens to the pan and let wilt for about 2 minutes.

In each serving bowl, place ½ cup Quinoa and top with sliced lamb and a few leaves of wilted greens. Finish with ¼ cup Coconut Milk Curry over the top. Garnish with fresh herbs and serve immediately.

**PER SERVING:** 660 calories, 49 grams fat, 24 grams saturated fat, 520 mg sodium, 31 grams carbohydrate (25 grams net carbs), 6 grams fiber, 3 grams sugar (0 added sugar), 30 grams protein

**GF**

## QUINOA

**Makes approximately 3 cups**

1 cup dry quinoa
2 cups unsalted vegetable stock
½ teaspoon sea salt
1 lime, zested
¼ cup coconut oil

In a pot over medium heat, combine quinoa, stock, and sea salt. Bring to a simmer then reduce heat to low. Cover with a lid and cook 15-20 minutes, or until quinoa is tender. Fluff with a fork and fold in the lime zest and coconut oil before serving.

## Nutrition Bite

Many perceive lamb as a high-fat, high-calorie food, but lamb *loin* is actually a leaner cut of meat.

## Cost Saver

Lamb loin is pricey. If you're not ready to shell out the bucks, you can use pork loin or beef tenderloin instead.

## HARISSA PASTE

**Makes 1 cup**

- 2 tablespoons cumin seed
- 2 tablespoons coriander seed
- 2 tablespoons black peppercorn
- 2 tablespoons caraway
- 2 tablespoons fenugreek
- 6 dry Thai chilis (or any dried chili peppers)
- 2 tablespoons curry powder
- 2 tablespoons paprika
- 2 tablespoons tomato paste
- 1 tablespoon light olive oil
- 6 inches of fresh ginger, peeled and minced
- 2 stalks lemongrass, minced
- 8 cloves garlic, minced

Preheat oven to 250 degrees. Spread cumin, coriander, black peppercorn, caraway, fenugreek, and Thai chilis onto a sheet pan and toast until lightly browned. Once cooled, grind into a powder using a coffee grinder or blender (or with a mortar and pestle) and mix with curry powder and paprika.

In a cast-iron skillet over medium heat, lightly heat tomato paste and oil for 3-5 minutes. Add toasted ground spices, ginger, lemongrass, and garlic to the pan and continue to heat for 4 minutes. Remove from heat and allow to cool, then place the mixture into a food processor and blend for 2 minutes. Store in an airtight container in the refrigerator.

## COCONUT MILK CURRY

**Makes approximately 2 cups**

- ¼ cup coconut oil
- ¼ yellow onion, minced
- 1 clove garlic, minced
- 1 tablespoon minced ginger
- 2-inch stalk lemongrass, minced
- 1 lime leaf, bruised (substitute fresh bay leaf and lime zest)
- ¼ teaspoon ground cumin
- ¼ teaspoon ground coriander
- ¼ teaspoon sea salt
- ¼ teaspoon freshly ground black pepper
- ¼ cup Harissa Paste
- 1 cup canned unsweetened coconut milk
- ½ cup thinly sliced cilantro

In a large pot over medium-low heat, mix together coconut oil and onion and sweat for 3 minutes. Stir in garlic, ginger, lemongrass, lime leaf, cumin, coriander, salt, pepper, and Harissa Paste. Continue to cook for 3 minutes. Add coconut milk and bring to a simmer, then immediately turn off the heat; do not boil. Add cilantro and steep for 30 minutes. Serve warm, though Maypop's Chef Michael recommends refrigerating for at least 12 hours to allow flavors to continue to steep.

## Time Saver /

Store-bought harissa paste is an easy shortcut if you're pressed for time.

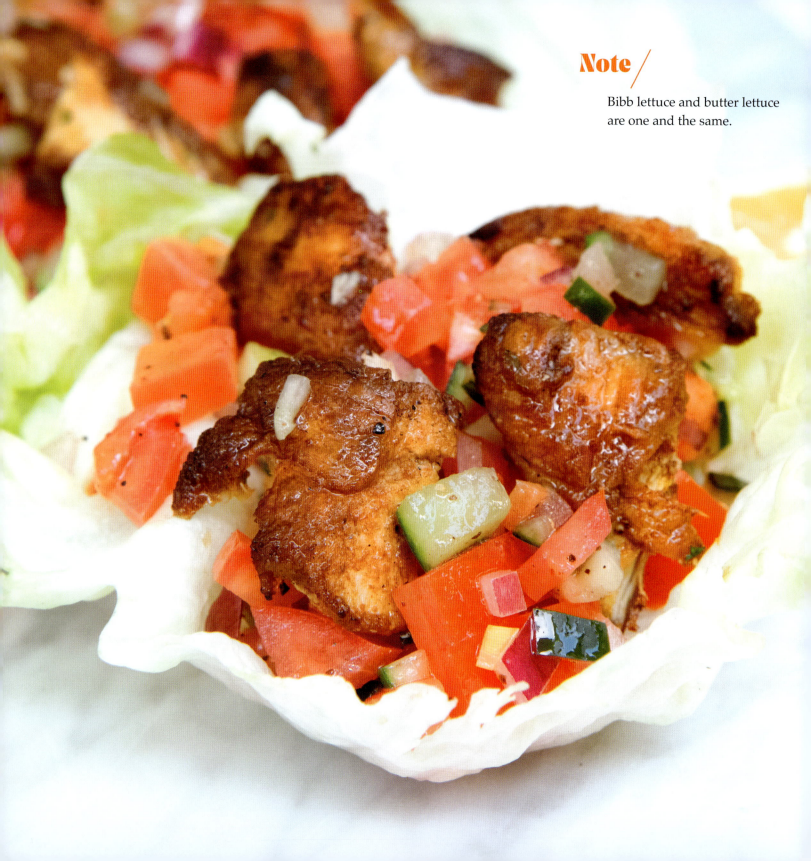

### Note

Bibb lettuce and butter lettuce are one and the same.

# Chicken Shawarma Lettuce Cups
## Attiki Bar & Grill

**Makes 6 servings**

Who says feeding a crowd has to be difficult? These savory and spicy lettuce cups work well in just about any setting. Marinating and grilling the chicken in advance makes for quick and easy assembly. For a casual atmosphere, guests can build their own lettuce cups with a do-it-yourself shawarma bar. If your event is more formal, serve the ready-made shawarma cups to your guests as a delightfully different amuse-bouche.

### For the Chicken

- 1 cup Attiki Chicken Shawarma Marinade (recipe follows)
- 2 pounds boneless skinless chicken breasts, cut into strips
- 1 teaspoon light olive oil
- ½ large red onion, thinly sliced
- ½ teaspoon sumac or lemon pepper seasoning

### For the Lettuce Cups

- 6 large Bibb lettuce leaves
- 1½ cups Chopped Mediterranean Salad (page 93)
- ⅓ cup Tahini (page 173)

Toss chicken with Attiki Chicken Shawarma Marinade in a large bowl. Cover and refrigerate for 3 hours.

Heat olive oil in a griddle or cast-iron skillet over medium heat. Sear chicken 4-5 minutes until charred on one side. Flip and grill the other side for 3-4 minutes, until chicken is cooked through. Add onion and cook until translucent. Sprinkle with sumac and remove from heat.

**Assemble the Lettuce Cups:** Pile chicken and onion into Bibb lettuce leaves. Top each with ¼ cup Chopped Mediterranean Salad and drizzle each with 1 tablespoon Tahini.

### ATTIKI CHICKEN SHAWARMA MARINADE

**Makes approximately 1 cup**

- ½ cup extra virgin olive oil
- ½ cup lemon juice
- 2 teaspoons paprika
- 2 teaspoons turmeric
- 2 teaspoons garlic powder
- 1 teaspoon ground cumin
- 1 teaspoon curry powder
- ⅛ teaspoon freshly ground black pepper
- ¼ tablespoon cayenne
- ½ teaspoon sea salt

Whisk together all ingredients until combined.

**PER SERVING:** 250 calories, 9 grams fat, 1.5 grams saturated fat, 150 mg sodium, 4 grams carbohydrate (3 grams net carbs), 1 gram fiber, 1 gram sugar (0 added sugar), 36 grams protein

GF, Low Carb

MAIN

## Serve It Up

We love this dish served appetizer style, with small-diced chicken on endive "spoons."

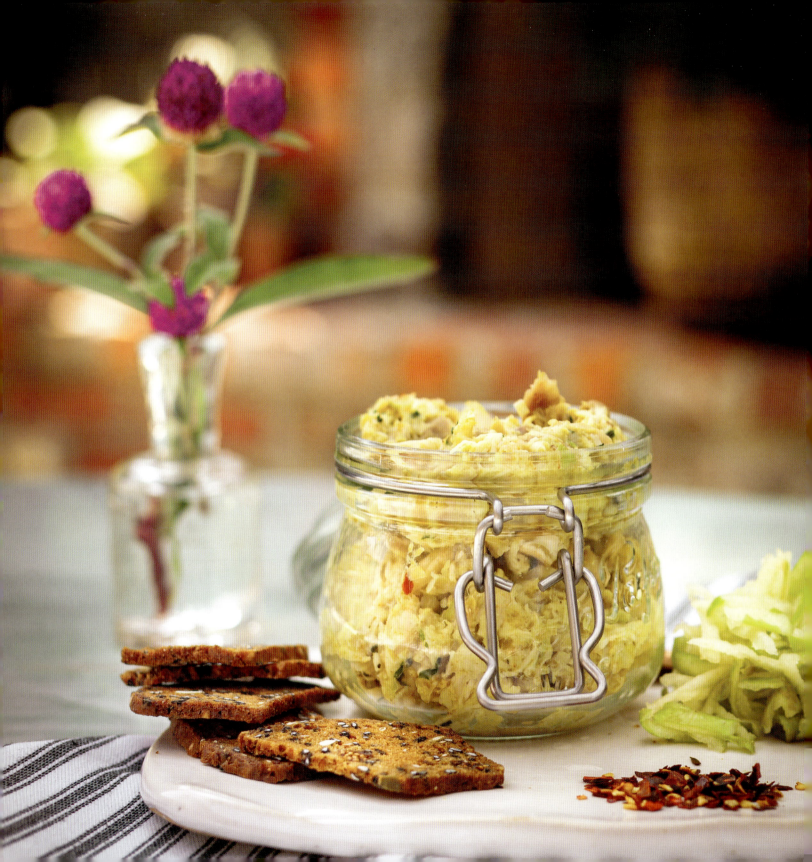

# Day-Brightening Curry Chicken Salad
## FUEL Café + Market

**Makes 6-8 servings**

As soon as we tasted this curry chicken salad by our FUEL Café Executive Chef Ryan Conn, it became one of those dishes we can't stop thinking about. As for the day-brightening part? We know that's a big statement, and we're comfortable standing behind it. Give it a try, share it, spread the love—and see for yourself.

1 whole chicken, roasted (or store-bought rotisserie chicken), to yield 4 cups pulled chicken
½ cup raw cashews, lightly toasted
1 green apple, grated
1 teaspoon chopped cilantro
1 batch of Mango Chutney (page 186)

Remove both the white and dark meat from the bone, hand-shredding and then roughly chopping any larger pieces; should be about 4 cups of pulled chicken, loosely packed.

In a large mixing bowl, combine the chicken, cashews, green apple, and cilantro. Slowly add the Mango Chutney and mix until evenly combined.

Serve on an Eat Fit croissant, grainy toast, atop mixed greens, or simply solo as it is. It's ready to eat right away—but Chef Ryan says (and we agree) it's even better after a few hours (or a day or so) in the fridge.

**PER SERVING:** 310 calories, 13 grams fat, 7 grams saturated fat, 490 mg sodium, 17 grams carbohydrate (14 grams net carbs), 3 grams fiber, 10 grams sugar (0 added sugar), 32 grams protein
GF, Low Carb

MAIN

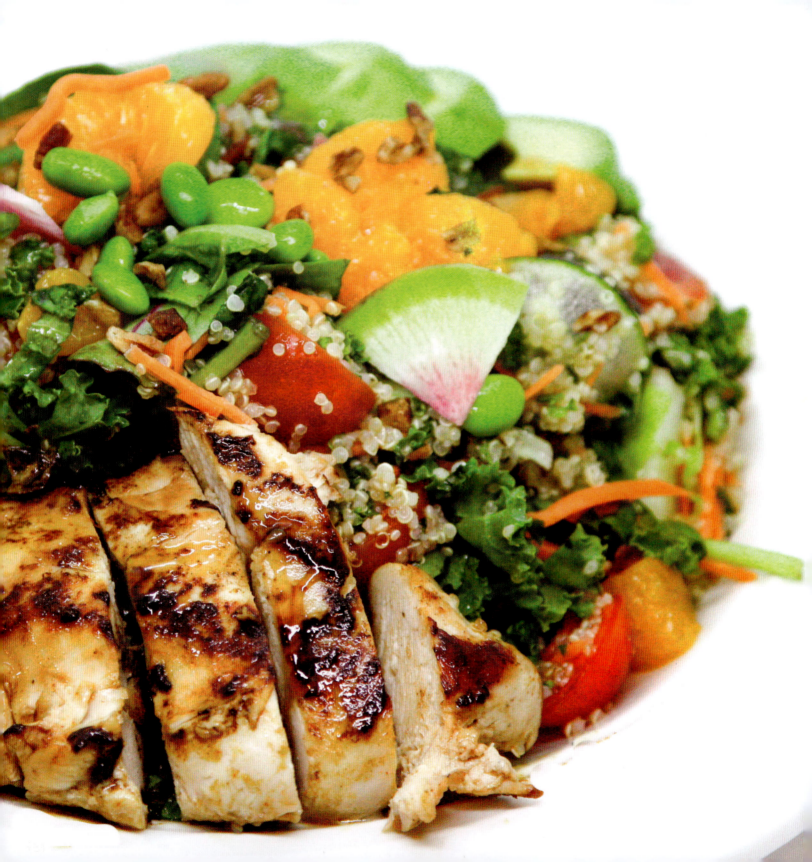

# Thai Quinoa + Kale Salad with Grilled Chicken
## Blue Line Sandwich Co.

**Makes 4 servings**

Two words: nutritional powerhouse. Boasting an impressive array of ingredients, this salad is an all-encompassing marvel, offering just the right balance of protein, fiber, and plant-based fats.

- ¼ cup Thai Chicken Marinade (recipe follows)
- 4 boneless, skinless chicken breasts, 6 ounces each
- 1 teaspoon light olive oil
- 3 cups chopped fresh kale
- 2 cups fresh baby spinach
- ¼ cup roughly chopped fresh cilantro
- ½ cup shredded carrot
- ½ cup satsuma segments
- ½ cup edamame, steamed and shelled
- 1 cup halved cherry or grape tomatoes
- ¼ cup toasted pecan pieces
- 1 cup cooked white quinoa
- 1 cup cooked red quinoa
- ½ cup Thai Peanut Dressing (page 176)
- 2 ripe avocados, diced

Marinate chicken in Thai Chicken Marinade. Heat griddle or cast-iron skillet over medium-high heat. Add oil to griddle or skillet and grill chicken for 5 minutes on each side, until chicken is cooked through. Remove from heat and slice into strips.

In a large mixing bowl, combine kale and the next 9 ingredients. Add Thai Peanut Dressing and toss until well-coated. Portion into serving bowls or plates, top with chicken breast, and garnish with avocado.

### THAI CHICKEN MARINADE

**Makes ¼ cup**

- 1 tablespoon seasoned rice vinegar
- 1½ garlic cloves, minced
- 1 tablespoon minced fresh ginger
- ½ tablespoon reduced sodium soy sauce
- ½ tablespoon toasted sesame seeds
- ½ teaspoon sesame oil
- 1 tablespoon light olive oil

Whisk together all ingredients until combined.

**PER SERVING:** 560 calories, 28 grams fat, 4.5 grams saturated fat, 330 mg sodium, 37 grams carbohydrate (28 grams net carbs), 9 grams fiber, 8 grams sugar (2 grams added sugar), 44 grams protein

## By the Way

Chef-owner Brad McGehee keeps this salad as close to home as possible, using homegrown kale, Louisiana satsumas (in place of oranges), and locally sourced pecans (in place of peanuts).

## Serve It Up

Red and white quinoa look really pretty in this dish, but any color quinoa can work.

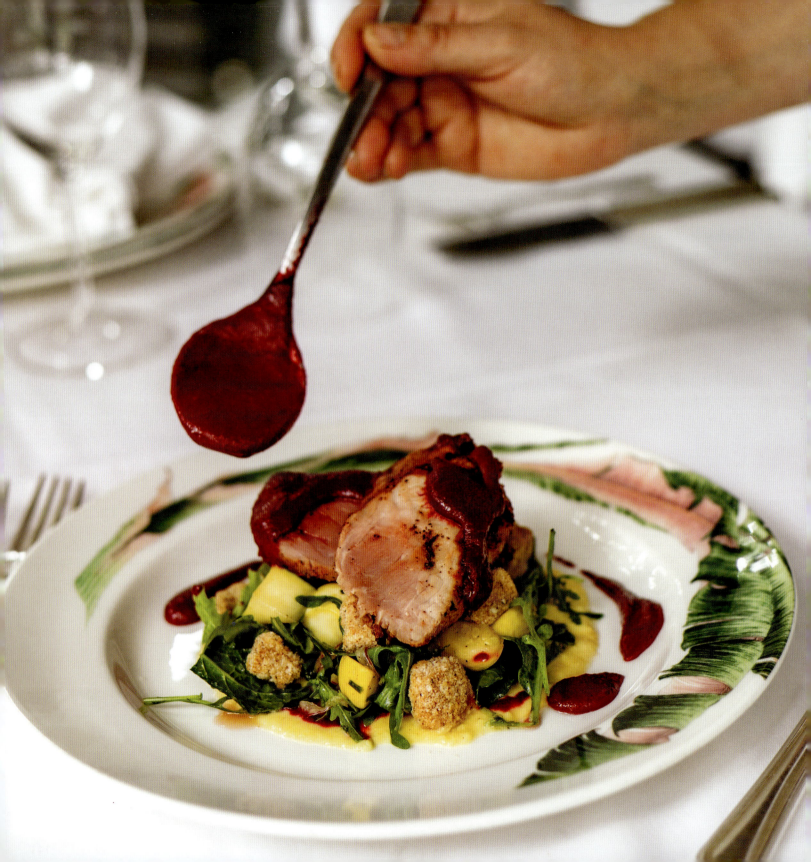

# Grilled Pork Tenderloin with Blueberry Beet Barbecue Sauce

## Commander's Palace

Chef Meg works her magic again, topping savory pork tenderloin with a gorgeous blueberry beet barbecue sauce and eggplant croutons. Trust us that you'll want to make extra sauce—it freezes well, and pairs perfectly with any lean meat or poultry.

**Makes 4 servings**

1 pork tenderloin, approximately 1½ pounds
1 teaspoon low-sodium Creole seasoning or Montreal steak seasoning
1 batch Sweet Corn Creole Cream Cheese (recipe follows)
1 batch Griddled Summer Squash and Tender Greens (page 90)
1 batch Eggplant Croutons (page 165)
½ cup Blueberry Beet Barbecue Sauce (page 185)

Season tenderloin and grill over medium heat for 8 to 10 minutes, until there are nice hash marks on each side. Let pork rest; cover with foil to keep warm.

Smear a tablespoon or so of the Sweet Corn Creole Cream Cheese on the base of a plate. Add half a cup of Griddled Summer Squash and Tender Greens Salad on top of smear. Slice pork tenderloin and place onto salad. Sprinkle a couple of spoonfuls of Eggplant Croutons around the salad. Drizzle two tablespoons of Blueberry Beet Barbecue Sauce over the top and serve.

## SWEET CORN CREOLE CREAM CHEESE
**Makes ½ cup**

1 ear of corn (or half a cup of corn kernels, roasted)
2 tablespoons Creole cream cheese (regular cream cheese if Creole style isn't available)
2 tablespoons buttermilk
1 teaspoon rice wine vinegar
Zest of ½ small lemon
Pinch of kosher salt
Pinch of white pepper

Roast corn in husk at 350 degrees for 15 minutes until golden brown and fragrant. Allow corn to cool. Clean corn from husk and cut kernels from cob. Place all ingredients in a blender, or use an immersion stick, and puree ingredients on high until smooth. Adjust seasoning to taste.

**PER SERVING:** 600 calories, 30 grams fat, 8 grams saturated fat, 810 mg sodium, 37 grams carbohydrate (28 grams net carbs), 9 grams fiber, 14 grams sugar (0 added sugar), 50 grams protein
**GF**

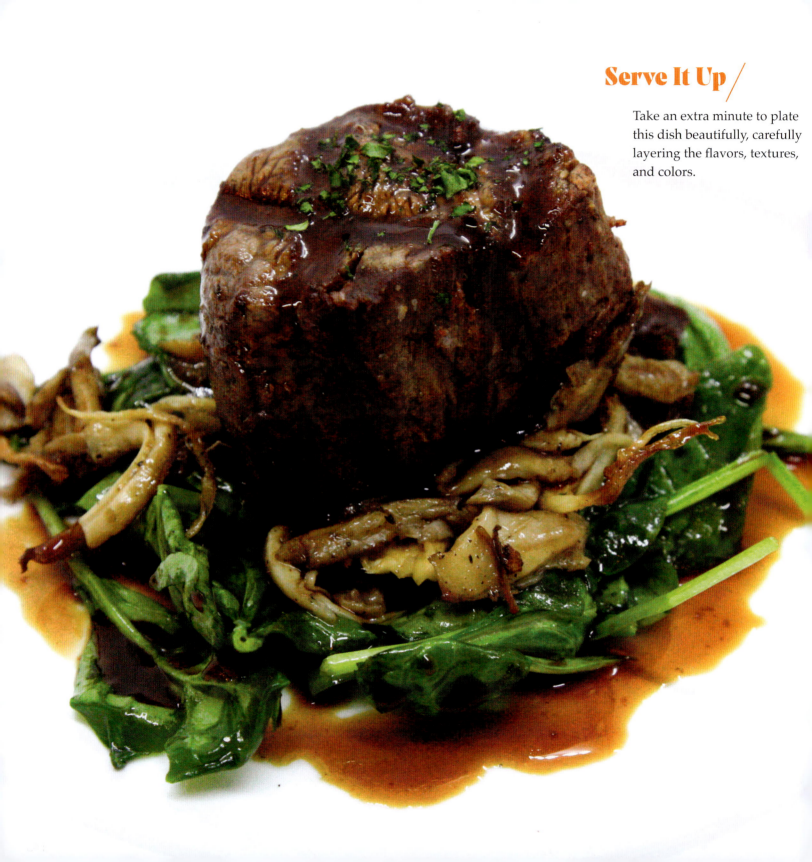

## Serve It Up /

Take an extra minute to plate this dish beautifully, carefully layering the flavors, textures, and colors.

# Petite Cartwright Filet
## Ye Olde College Inn

**Makes 4 servings**

If this steak were Batman, it wouldn't need a Robin (sorry, potato). Its rich demi-glace sauce adds a dimension of flavor we miss out on when grilling at home.

- 4 beef filets, 6 ounces each
- ½ teaspoon sea salt, divided
- 1 teaspoon freshly ground black pepper, divided
- 3 tablespoons light olive oil, divided
- ½ cup Demi-Glace (recipe follows)
- 3 cups thinly sliced or torn mushrooms
- 1 tablespoon minced garlic
- 3 thyme sprigs
- ¼ cup dry red wine
- 6 cups baby spinach
- 2 teaspoons chopped fresh parsley

Season each filet with a pinch each of salt and pepper and coat with 2 tablespoons olive oil. Grill filets on high heat for 3 minutes per side for medium rare and 4-5 minutes per side for medium. Let rest for 5 minutes before slicing. Meanwhile, in a small saucepan, slowly heat the Demi-Glace.

In a large skillet over high heat, sauté mushrooms in remaining oil until nicely browned. Add garlic and remaining salt and pepper and cook for 30 seconds. Add thyme and red wine to deglaze the pan. Add spinach and cook until wilted, stirring constantly. To serve, portion the spinach and mushroom mixture onto each plate, top with filet, drizzle with Demi-Glace, and garnish with parsley.

## DEMI-GLACE

**Makes approximately 3 quarts**

- ½ bottle Cabernet Sauvignon (375 ml)
- 5 pounds veal or beef bones
- 2½ gallons water
- 8 black peppercorns
- 1 bunch fresh parsley
- 1 bay leaf
- 7 sprigs thyme
- 2 yellow onions, cut into quarters
- 2 carrots, cut into chunks
- 4 celery stalks, cut into 3-inch pieces
- 1 teaspoon sea salt

Combine all ingredients in a large pot and cover with water. Bring to a boil and reduce to a simmer. Cook for 24 hours over low heat.

**PER SERVING:** 430 calories, 19 grams fat, 7 grams saturated fat, 310 mg sodium, 5 grams carbohydrate (3 grams net carbs), 2 grams fiber, 1 gram sugar (0 added sugar), 55 grams protein

**GF, Low Carb**

## Nutrition Bite

Although filet seems ultra-decadent, it's a lean cut of beef that's relatively low in animal saturated fat.

## Time Saver

Streamline the 24-hour Demi-Glace with 4 quarts unsalted stock in place of water. Add ½ bottle of red wine and Demi-Glace vegetables. Bring to a boil then reduce heat and simmer for several hours until reduced by half. Strain out the vegetables, add the remaining ½ bottle of wine, and return to a boil. Reduce heat and simmer for several hours until reduced by half.

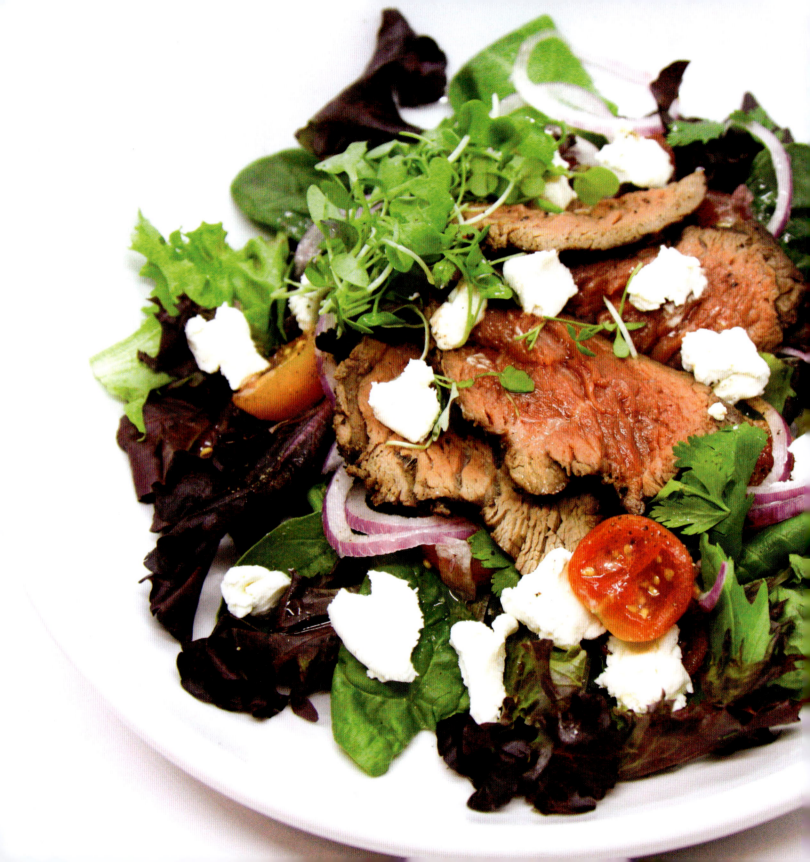

# Grilled Steak Salad with Red Wine Vinaigrette
## *Kingfish*

**Makes 4 servings**

When we learn that steak dishes are Eat Fit approved, we smile. When we learn that steak dishes served with goat cheese are Eat Fit approved, we throw a grand parade. Typically considered bad boys on the health front, steak and cheese don't have to be omitted from our diets altogether. Using lean beef paired with good quality cheese (just don't be too grabby here) makes it easy to enjoy two of life's simple indulgences.

### Grilled Steak

4 filets mignons, 6 ounces each
2 tablespoons light olive oil
¼ teaspoon sea salt
¼ teaspoon freshly ground black pepper

### Salad

4 cups spring mix
¼ red onion, thinly sliced
½ cup Red Wine Vinaigrette (page 178)
¼ teaspoon sea salt
⅛ teaspoon freshly ground black pepper
½ cup halved cherry tomatoes
2 tablespoons crumbled goat cheese
¼ cup microgreens for garnish

**Grill the Steak:** Allow filets to sit at room temperature for 30 minutes. Toss with oil and season with salt and pepper. Place on a hot grill and cook on both sides until filets reach desired temperature. Remove from heat and set aside.

**Assemble the Salad:** Combine spring mix, onion, vinaigrette, salt, and pepper in a large bowl and toss to combine. Divide salad onto 4 plates. Thinly slice steak against the grain and fan across salad. Top with tomatoes and goat cheese, garnish with microgreens, and serve.

**PER SERVING:** 550 calories, 32 grams fat, 9 grams saturated fat, 610 mg sodium, 8 grams carbohydrate (5 grams net carbs), 3 grams fiber, 3 grams sugar (0 added sugar), 56 grams protein

GF, Low Carb

## Chef Tip /

Rinse red onions under cold water to remove bitterness.

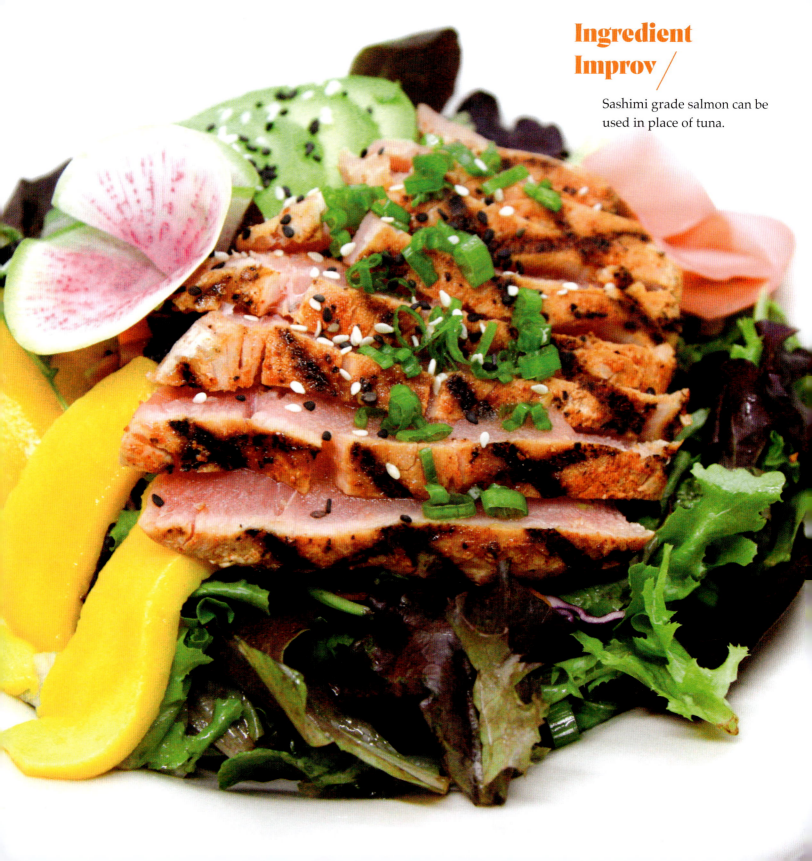

## Ingredient Improv /

Sashimi grade salmon can be used in place of tuna.

# Mango Tuna Sashimi Salad
## *Superior Grill*

**Makes 4 servings**

Superior Grill's Mango Tuna Sashimi Salad could not be more gorgeous. Its colorful flavors and variety of textures create a fiesta for the taste buds.

**8 cups spring mix**
**½ cup Ginger Dressing (page 171)**
**4 sushi grade tuna fillets, 6 ounces each**
**½ avocado, thinly sliced**
**½ mango, thinly sliced**
**¼ cup finely chopped fresh cilantro**

Toss spring mix in Ginger Dressing and set aside.

Sear tuna on grill or cast-iron skillet over high heat for 1 minute on each side or until fish reaches desired temperature. Set aside and allow to rest for 2 minutes.

Thinly slice tuna against the grain. Plate the dressed greens and top with tuna, avocado, and mango slices. Garnish with cilantro and serve.

**PER SERVING:** 310 calories, 11 grams fat, 2.5 grams saturated fat, 290 mg sodium, 12 grams carbohydrate (9 grams net carbs), 3 grams fiber, 6 grams sugar (0 added sugar), 41 grams protein
LOW CARB

## Love It Later

Make extra Ginger Dressing to spice up your next plain ol' chicken dish.

## Ingredient Improv

Don't have mango? Use fresh pineapple or green apple for sweetness and color contrast.

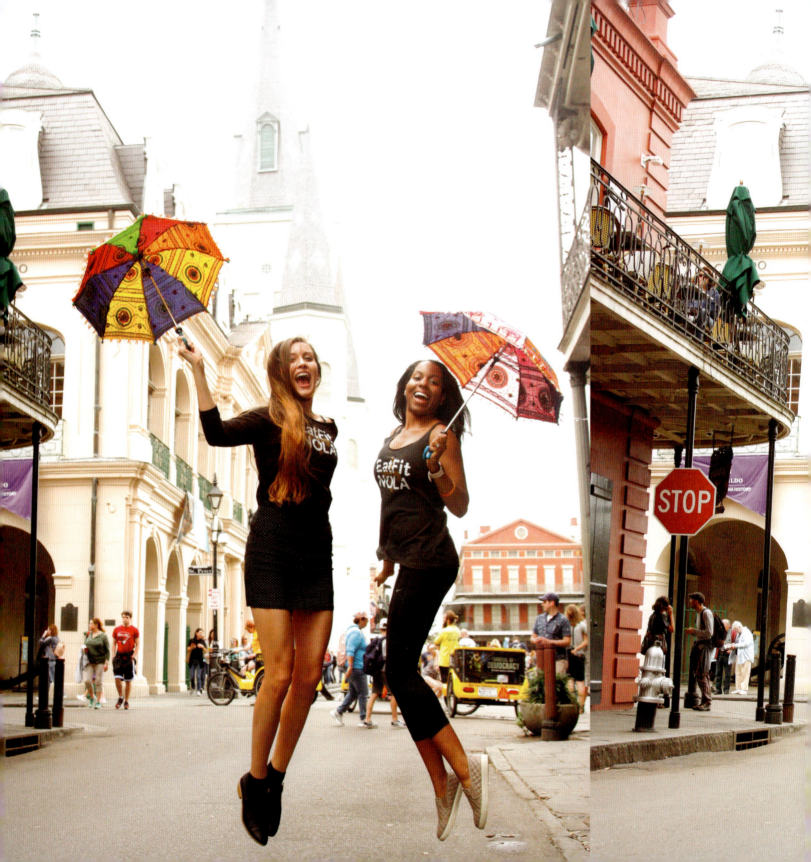

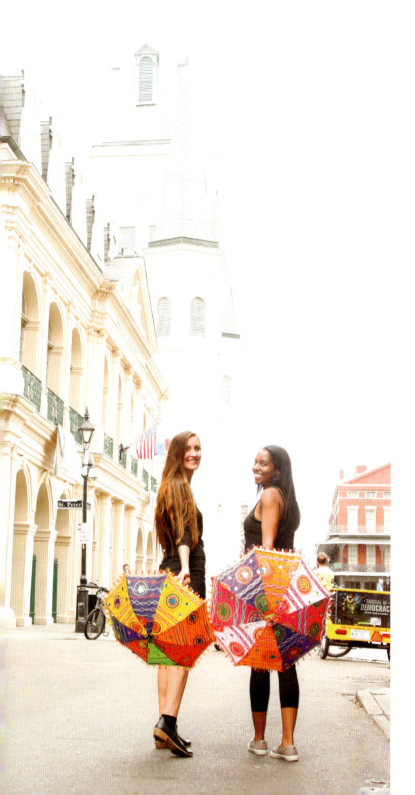

# 5
# LAGNIAPPE
## *Accompaniments + Sides*

We refuse to settle for the mundane, the unimaginative, and the I-am-just-eating-this-because-it's-what's-here type of food. We look at meals as opportunities for culinary creations to nourish our bodies, our minds, and our souls. We spice up our favorite recipes NOLA-style with uncomplicated yet gratifying accompaniments and sides that harmonize beautifully with the main dishes to create the music that is our food.

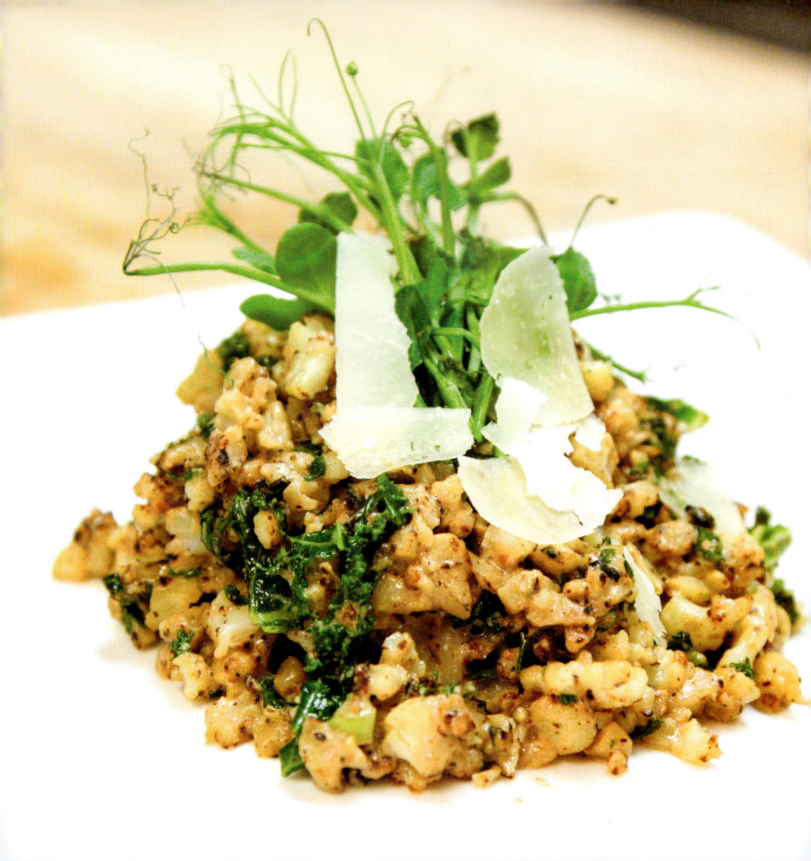

# Wilted Kale + Roasted Cauliflower "Risotto"

*Dakota Restaurant*

**Makes 6 servings**

Cauliflower once again saves the day! We love this starchless risotto paired with any protein.

1 tablespoon light olive oil
2 tablespoons minced garlic
2 cups grated raw cauliflower or store-bought riced cauliflower
2 cups chopped raw kale
¼ teaspoon sea salt
1½ teaspoons black pepper
½ cup unsalted vegetable broth
½ cup 2% plain Greek yogurt
½ teaspoon chopped fresh basil
½ teaspoon chopped fresh thyme
1 teaspoon chopped fresh parsley
¼ cup Parmesan Reggiano
1 tablespoon butter

In a medium skillet over high heat, heat oil until almost smoking. Add garlic and cauliflower and sauté until lightly caramelized. Reduce heat to medium. Add kale and season with salt and pepper. Cook until kale is partially wilted. Stir in broth, yogurt, basil, thyme, and parsley. Simmer until heated through. Remove from heat and fold in Parmesan Reggiano and butter. Serve immediately.

**PER SERVING:** 90 calories, 6 grams fat, 2.5 grams saturated fat, 160 mg sodium, 5 grams carbohydrate (4 grams net carbs), 1 gram fiber, 1 gram sugar (0 added sugar), 5 grams protein

GF, Low Carb, Vegetarian

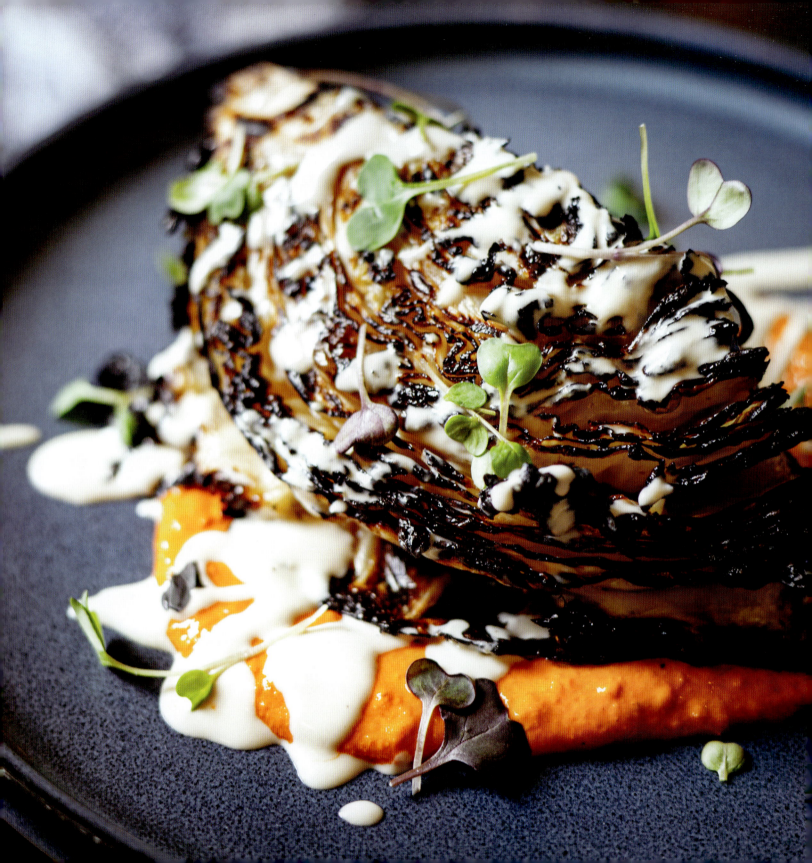

# Charred Cabbage with Hazelnut Muhammara and Tahini
## *Saba*

**Makes 4 plates (8 servings)**

It's a rare thing for cabbage to be just so beautiful. And the visual appeal of this shared plate by Alon Shaya is only the beginning. Each bite is a sensory celebration of flavors and textures, the lightly-charred-yet-buttery-soft cabbage paired with the savory, smoky muhammara and delicate tahini drizzle.

- 2 quarts water
- ½ cup plus 3 tablespoons extra-virgin olive oil, divided
- 2 tablespoons plus 1 teaspoon kosher salt, divided
- ½ cup orange juice
- ½ cup rice wine vinegar, preferably seasoned
- 2 tablespoons sugar
- 2 cloves garlic
- 1 jalapeño, seeds and pith (membrane around the seeds) removed, sliced
- 1 star anise pod
- 1 lemon, zested
- 1 medium head green cabbage
- 1 cup Muhammara (page 174)
- ¼ cup Tahini (page 173)
- ¼ cup chopped hazelnuts for garnish
- Handful of microgreens for garnish

In a deep pot that is not too wide and just large enough to hold a head of cabbage as snugly as possible, add water, half cup of olive oil, 2 tablespoons salt, plus orange juice, rice wine vinegar, sugar, garlic, jalapeño, star anise, and lemon zest. Bring to a boil, then reduce heat to medium. Simmer for 10-15 minutes.

Meanwhile, trim any tough outer leaves from cabbage. Halve it lengthwise. Taste the broth—when it's been infused with the jalapeño and garlic, carefully lower the cabbage halves into the pot (a couple of large spoons can help manipulate it and minimize splashing).

Reduce heat to low and cover. After 30 minutes, check the tenderness. The cabbage is ready when it's easily pierced with a knife but still resists slightly. If, after an hour, it's still a bit too firm, rotate it again, cover, and continue to cook, checking every 5 to 10 minutes until it's ready. Depending on the size of cabbage, cooking can take up to 1½ hours—the perfect amount of time to make matbucha.

With a slotted spoon or a strainer, remove cabbage from the pot and transfer to a rimmed baking sheet. Allow to cool slightly. Strain and reserve the broth for future use—such as a soup base—if desired. Meanwhile, heat oven broiler with rack in the upper-middle position.

Leaving stem ends intact, cut cabbage halves again, lengthwise, essentially quartering the cabbage. Drain away any excess liquid. Remove leaves that are so soft they are falling off. Place each wedge on a baking sheet, curved (outer) side down. Brush or drizzle with two tablespoons of olive oil, and sprinkle with remaining salt.

Broil 10-12 minutes, rotating baking sheet halfway through, until charred all along edges—this is what adds flavor and interest to an otherwise overlooked vegetable.

To serve, smear a quarter cup or so of Muhammara onto each plate. Top with charred cabbage quarter, drizzle with olive oil and a tablespoon of Tahini. Garnish with a tablespoon of chopped hazelnuts and microgreens.

PER SERVING: 190 calories, 14 grams fat, 1.5 grams saturated fat, 110 mg sodium, 14 grams carbohydrate (9 grams net carbs), 5 grams fiber, 7 grams sugar (0 added sugar), 4 grams protein
GF, Low Carb, Vegan, Low Sodium

# Brussels + Broccoli Mash
## Mestizo Louisiana Mexican Cuisine

**Makes 4 servings**

Steamed, roasted, grilled, sautéed, or even raw, broccoli and Brussels are highly nutritious vegetables that we think should be prominently featured on everyone's regular menu. Mestizo offers this creative twist on both that will likely have you reaching for seconds.

- 1 cup broccoli florets, cut into small pieces
- 1 cup Brussels sprouts, quartered
- 1 teaspoon red pepper flakes
- 2 cloves garlic, minced
- 4 tomatillos, quartered
- ½ cup diced white onion
- ½ teaspoon sea salt
- ½ teaspoon freshly ground black pepper
- 1 tablespoon light olive oil
- ¾ cup 2% plain Greek yogurt

Preheat oven to 400 degrees. Blanch broccoli and Brussels sprouts in boiling water for 3 minutes then submerge into ice water to stop the cooking.

On a sheet pan, spread blanched vegetables, red pepper flakes, garlic, tomatillos, onion, salt, and pepper. Drizzle with oil, then toss to coat. Roast for 25 minutes, flipping once or twice mid-way through.

Transfer roasted vegetables to a bowl and mash with the back of a serving spoon. Stir in yogurt to form a creamy, dip-like consistency. Serve warm, with thick-sliced carrots, red and yellow peppers, or whole-grain crostini.

PER SERVING: 110 calories, 5 grams fat, 1 gram saturated fat, 125 mg sodium, 12 grams carbohydrate (8 grams net carbs), 4 grams fiber, 5 grams sugar (0 added sugar), 7 grams protein
GF, Low Carb, Vegetarian, Low Sodium

## Ingredient Improv

Can't find tomatillos? Use green tomatoes (seeds removed) with a squeeze of lime instead.

## Serve It Up

Serve this dish in place of a starchy side like grits, polenta, or mashed potatoes.

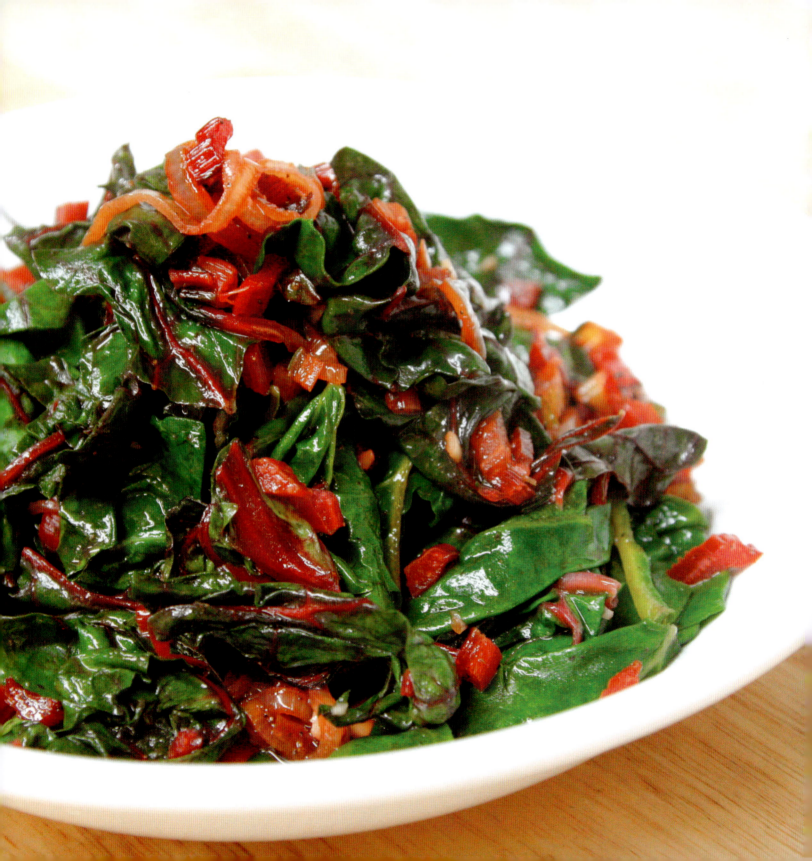

# Sautéed Swiss Chard
## Blue Dog Café

**Makes 4 servings**

The Blue Dog Café prepares this nutrient-packed side dish using locally sourced ingredients.

**2 pounds fresh Swiss chard**
**3 tablespoons cold-pressed pecan oil**
**3 cloves fresh garlic, minced**
**1 ounce white wine (such as Chardonnay)**
**1 lemon, juiced**
**Dash of sea salt (optional)**
**Dash of freshly ground black pepper**

Prepare Swiss chard by separating the leaves from the stems. Set aside the leaves and small dice the stems.

In a large sauté pan over medium-high heat, sauté the diced stems in oil for 1 minute. Once stems are tender, add the leaves, toss, and sauté for 30 seconds. Add garlic, toss, and sauté 30 seconds. Deglaze with white wine and cook for another 30 seconds. Remove pan from heat and add lemon juice, salt, and black pepper. Serve warm.

**PER SERVING:** 150 calories, 11 grams fat, 1.5 grams saturated fat, 480 mg sodium, 10 grams carbohydrate (6 grams net carbs), 4 grams fiber, 3 grams sugar (0 added sugar), 4 grams protein
 GF, Low Carb, Vegan

LAGNIAPPE

## By the Way

If pecan oil isn't readily available at your supermarket, just use extra virgin olive oil instead.

# Butternut Squash Hash
## Café Vermilionville

**Makes 4 servings**

Fresh and colorful, this dish is a cinch to make.

**1 large butternut squash, cubed**
**2 tablespoons light olive oil, divided**
**1 medium yellow summer squash, cubed**
**1 medium zucchini, cubed**
**½ medium red bell pepper, cubed**
**¼ medium red onion, cubed**
**½ teaspoon sea salt**
**Pinch of freshly ground black pepper**

Preheat oven to 350 degrees. Toss butternut squash in 1 tablespoon oil. Spread onto baking sheet lined with foil and roast in oven until soft, approximately 30-40 minutes, turning several times.

Heat remaining 1 tablespoon oil in a saucepan over medium-high heat. Add the summer squash, zucchini, bell pepper, and red onion, and cook for about 7 minutes. Add roasted butternut squash and cook for another 2-3 minutes, until fork-tender. Season with salt and pepper and sauté until lightly browned. Serve immediately.

**PER SERVING:** 150 calories, 7 grams fat, 1 gram saturated fat, 180 mg sodium, 21 grams carbohydrate (17 grams net carbs), 4 grams fiber, 6 grams sugar (0 added sugar), 3 grams protein
**GF, Vegan**

## Nutrition Bite

This dish provides nearly a day's worth of vitamins A and C.

# Roasted Pepper Quinoa Pilaf
## Ye Olde College Inn

**Makes 6 servings**

Think rice pilaf, but better for you.

1 red bell pepper
1 green bell pepper
2 tablespoons light olive oil
2 shallots, minced
4 garlic cloves, minced
1 cup dry quinoa
5 sprigs fresh thyme
4 cups unsalted vegetable broth
¼ teaspoon sea salt
¼ teaspoon ground black pepper

Roast peppers over an open flame until charred black all around. Immediately place charred peppers in a mixing bowl and cover to steam and loosen skin. Once the peppers have cooled, remove the skin, stem, and seeds. Medium dice the roasted peppers and set aside.

In a medium pot over medium heat, combine olive oil, shallots, and roasted peppers and cook for 2-3 minutes. Add the garlic and stir for 30 seconds. Mix in the quinoa and stir until coated. Add thyme, broth, salt, and pepper then increase heat to high and bring to a boil. Once boiling, reduce heat to low and cover tightly. Simmer for 20 minutes. Remove from heat and let stand covered for 5 minutes. Fluff with a fork and serve.

**PER SERVING:** 110 calories, 5 grams fat, 1 gram saturated fat, 150 mg sodium, 12 grams carbohydrate (10 grams net carbs), 2 grams fiber, 3 grams sugar (0 added sugar), 5 grams protein
GF, Low Carb, Vegan

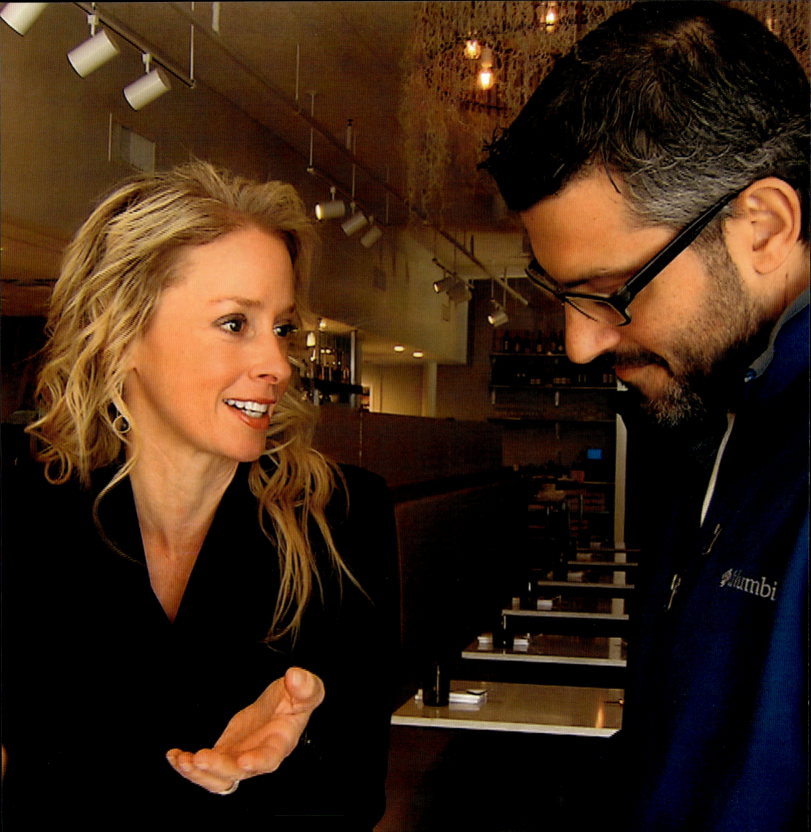

# White Beans
## Chef Carl Schaubhut

**Makes 8 servings**

Throughout Bayou Country, white beans are served as side dishes or entrées and devoured by friends and families around the dinner table. Chef Carl creates a delicious Eat Fit version of this Southern comfort food without the traditional salt and animal fat.

1 pound white beans, soaked overnight and drained
2 yellow onions, diced
2 carrots, peeled and diced
3 ribs celery, diced
1 tablespoon minced garlic
3 bay leaves
2 thyme sprigs

**For the Seasoning**
½ teaspoon sea salt
1 teaspoon ground black pepper
2 tablespoons Lea & Perrins Worcestershire sauce
2 tablespoons hot sauce
2 tablespoons Steen's cane vinegar
1 tablespoon miso

After soaking beans overnight, combine beans, onions, carrots, celery, and garlic in a large pot. Place bay leaves and thyme sprigs into a sachet and add to beans. Cover with cold water and bring to a boil. Skim off and discard any foam on the surface. Reduce to a simmer over low heat, cover, and cook until white beans are tender, about 2 hours (up to 4 hours if you like them really soft). Remove lid and simmer uncovered for 30-45 minutes to cook off any excess liquid.

Once beans are tender, remove the sachet and puree half of the beans in a food processor. Return the pureed beans to the pot and add the seasoning ingredients. Stir to combine. Serve warm.

**PER SERVING:** 110 calories, 0.5 grams fat, 0 saturated fat, 260 mg sodium, 22 grams carbohydrate (14 grams net carbs), 8 grams fiber, 3 grams sugar (0 added sugar), 6 grams protein

## Chef Tip

A seasoning sachet is easily made by filling cheesecloth with herbs and spices. Tie into a bundle with butcher's twine with the other end tied to the handle of the pot so that it can easily be removed after cooking.

> "We're not telling people to stay away from their favorite foods, we're actually offering healthy dishes for them so they don't even have to think about it."
> —Chef Carl Schaubhut

Molly and Chef Carl (*Courtesy WYES-TV Good Eating . . . Good Health*).

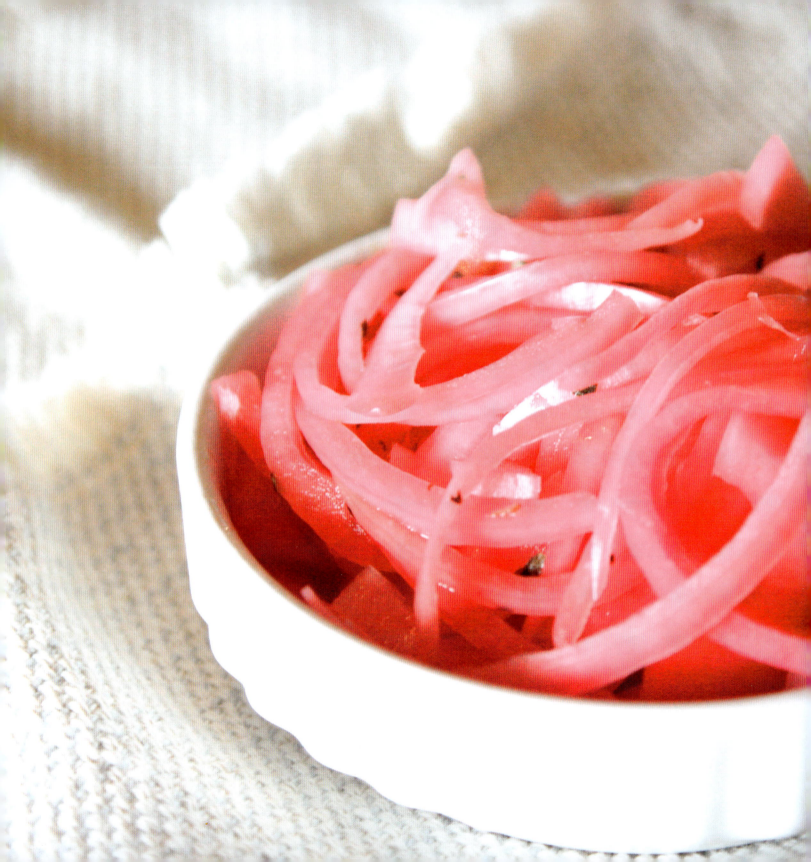

# Pickled Red Onions
## Eat Fit Collection

**Makes 8 servings**

Our Eat Fit restaurants collectively have about 200 different variations of pickled onions. Okay, maybe not quite that many, but it's a lot. We've streamlined them into one simple, low-calorie, low-sodium version here.

½ red onion, sliced
1 teaspoon Swerve Granular
1 pinch black pepper
2 cups apple cider vinegar or rice wine vinegar

In a medium bowl, combine onion, Swerve, black pepper, and vinegar. Soak for at least 1 hour. Refrigerate for up to 3 days.

PER SERVING: 0 calories, 0 fat, 0 saturated fat, 0 sodium, 0 carbohydrate (0 net carb), 0 fiber, 0 sugar, 0 protein

GF, Vegan, Low Carb, Low Sodium

### By the Way

This recipe can be used to make pickled red cabbage (or any other type of pickled vegetable). It's the same ratio, just substitute red cabbage for the onion.

# Ginger Pickled Mirliton
## Commander's Palace

**Makes approximately 2 cups**

¼ cup rice wine vinegar
2 tablespoons Swerve Granular
2 tablespoons white wine
1 tablespoon minced ginger
½ teaspoon mustard seeds
½ teaspoon white peppercorns
⅛ teaspoon ground cinnamon
⅛ teaspoon ground allspice
⅛ teaspoon ground nutmeg
⅛ teaspoon ground clove
¼ teaspoon sea salt
1 mirliton, deseeded and cut into ½-inch matchsticks
½ teaspoon grenadine

In a medium pot, combine all ingredients except mirliton and grenadine. Bring to a boil then reduce to a simmer for 5 minutes. Place mirliton in a shallow bowl and cover with mixture. Make sure mirliton is fully submerged. Add grenadine. Cool completely and refrigerate. Best if made about a week in advance.

PER TABLESPOON: 0 calories, 0 fat, 0 saturated fat, 10 mg sodium, <1 gram carbohydrate (<1 gram net carb), 0 fiber, 0 sugar, 0 protein

GF, Vegan, Low Carb, Low Sodium

### gren * a * dine

If you don't have grenadine on hand, use pomegranate juice or beet juice (or add just a few cubes of fresh beets) for a similar color. To thicken, heat in a saucepan over medium heat until reduced to a syrupy consistency.

# Beet Medallions
## Commander's Palace

**Makes 12 servings**

These thin, savory rounds add visual interest and appeal to our favorite soups and salads.

**2 large golden beets**
**½ teaspoon sea salt**
**Pinch of freshly ground black pepper**
**¼ cup chopped chives**
**¼ cup chopped fresh parsley leaves**

Preheat oven to 200 degrees. With a mandolin or very sharp knife, shave golden beets into very thin round chips. Lay flat on parchment-lined sheet pan and sprinkle with salt and pepper. Dehydrate in oven for 30 minutes. Garnish with chives and parsley.

PER SERVING: 5 calories, 0 fat, 0 saturated fat, 65 mg sodium, 1 gram carbohydrate (1 gram net carb), 0 fiber, <1 gram sugar (0 added sugar), 0 protein
GF, Low Carb, Vegan, Low Sodium

# Roasted Mushrooms
## SoBou

**Makes 4 servings**

Roasted mushrooms can be used as a meat replacement. Try substituting half of the ground beef in your next meat sauce or burger with mushrooms.

**2 cups chopped oyster mushrooms (substitute baby portobellos)**
**½ cup chopped fresh oregano**
**½ cup chopped fresh thyme**

Preheat oven to 350 degrees. Toss mushrooms with herbs, garlic, and olive oil. Spread evenly on a baking pan and roast for 10 minutes.

PER SERVING: 90 calories, 7 grams fat, 1 gram saturated fat, 15 mg sodium, 6 grams carbohydrate (4 grams net carbs), 2 grams fiber, <1 gram sugar (0 added sugar), 2 grams protein
GF, Low Carb, Vegan, Low Sodium

# Eggplant Croutons
## Commander's Palace

**Makes 1½ cups**

Chef Meg created these little cubes of breaded eggplant to complement the Pork Tenderloin with Blueberry Beet BBQ Sauce. We also think they're pretty fantastic dipped into a bit of marinara sauce or sliced a little larger to serve as eggplant "fries."

- 1 small eggplant
- 2 teaspoons kosher salt, divided
- 1 cup almond flour
- 1 tablespoon onion powder
- 1 tablespoon garlic powder
- 1 teaspoon red pepper flakes
- 1 tablespoon chopped fresh thyme (or 1 teaspoon dried)
- 1 tablespoon chopped parsley (or 1 teaspoon dried)
- 3 egg whites

Preheat oven to 350 degrees. Peel eggplant and cut into half-inch cubes. Sprinkle with teaspoon of salt and set aside for 30 minutes, to pull out moisture. Rinse well to remove excess salt. Pat dry.

In a mixing bowl, combine almond flour, onion powder, garlic powder, red pepper flakes, teaspoon of salt, thyme, and parsley, stirring until evenly mixed.

Whisk egg whites in a small bowl. Dredge eggplant in the whites, allowing excess to drip off, then toss into seasoned almond flour. Place battered eggplant cubes onto parchment-lined sheet tray. Roast 15 to 20 minutes, turning over midway through. Bake until golden.

PER SERVING: (2 tablespoons): 40 calories, 2 grams fat, 0 saturated fat, 70 mg sodium, 4 grams carbohydrate (3 grams net carbs), 1 gram fiber, 1 gram sugar (0 added sugar), 2 grams protein

GF, Low Carb, Vegetarian, Low Sodium

# Sambal Vegetable Stir Fry
## Commander's Palace

**Makes 4 servings**

This kicked-up stir fry has a hint of sweet and a lot of spice.

1 spaghetti squash
2 garlic cloves, minced
1 shallot, minced
½ red bell pepper, brunoised
1 teaspoon sesame oil
¼ teaspoon Sambal chili sauce
1 cup shiitake mushrooms, stemmed and julienned (substitute baby portobellos)
1 teaspoon reduced sodium soy sauce
1 cup packed pea shoots
¼ cup green onions, biased cut

Preheat oven to 350 degrees. Cut spaghetti squash in half lengthwise. Scoop out seeds and discard. Place squash skin side up on roasting pan. Pour 1 cup water into bottom of pan. Roast for 20 minutes, until fork tender. Remove from oven, flip skin side down, and cool on cooling rack. When cool enough to handle, scrape out squash with a fork; it should come out in strands like al dente pasta. Set aside.

In a large sauté pan over medium heat, sauté garlic, shallot, and bell pepper in sesame oil. Stir in chili sauce, squash, and mushrooms. Cook until squash is warmed through and mushrooms are slightly wilted. Add soy sauce, pea shoots, and green onions. Heat until the shoots are wilted.

**PER SERVING:** 100 calories, 2 grams fat, 0 saturated fat, 110 mg sodium, 20 grams carbohydrate (16 grams net carbs), 7 grams sugar (0 added sugar), 4 grams protein

VEGAN, LOW SODIUM

# Candied Walnuts
## English Tea Room

This recipe is one of our go-to favorites—it's even perfect for holiday gifting. We also use it to make Eat Fit candied cashews, pecans, macadamias, you name it. And if you're looking for a vegan option, just use coconut oil in place of butter.

**Makes 1 cup**

2 tablespoons butter (or coconut oil)
1 cup chopped walnuts
2 tablespoons Swerve Granular
¼ teaspoon ground cinnamon
⅛ teaspoon Tony Chachere's Cajun seasoning
2 tablespoons Swerve Brown Sugar Replacer

Melt butter in a saucepan over medium heat. Once melted, add walnuts to pan and coat. Sprinkle with Swerve Granular, cinnamon, and Tony Chachere's. Stir until caramelized. Remove from heat, spread onto parchment paper and separate. Sprinkle with Swerve Brown Sugar Replacer. Allow to fully cool before serving.

PER SERVING: 60 calories, 6 grams fat, 1 gram saturated fat, 10 mg sodium, 1 gram carbohydrate, 0 fiber, 0 sugar, 1 gram protein
GF, Low Carb, Vegetarian, Low Sodium

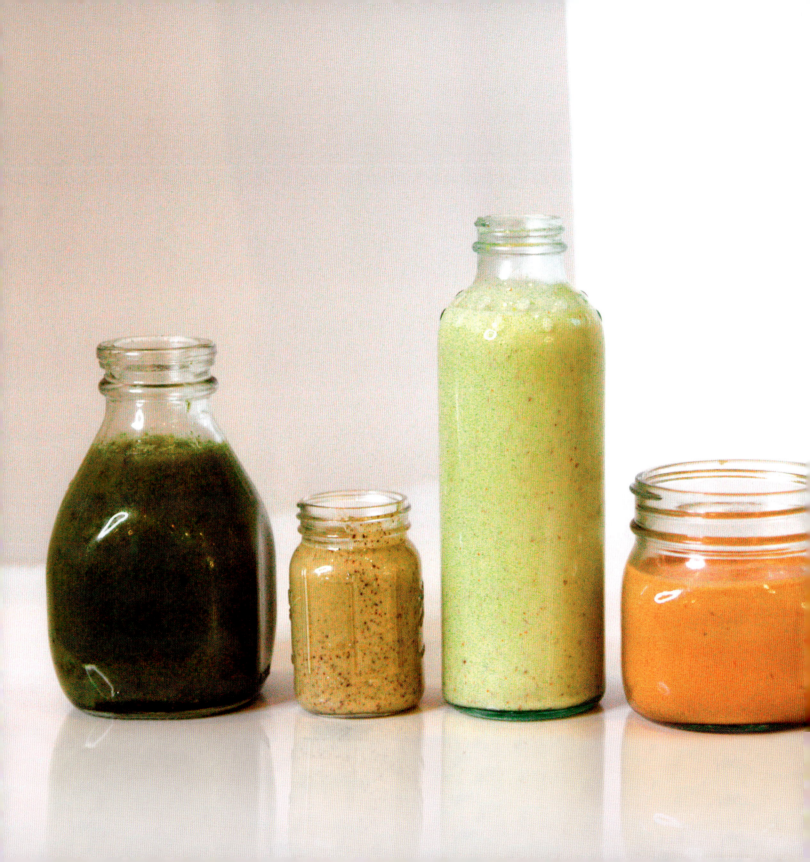

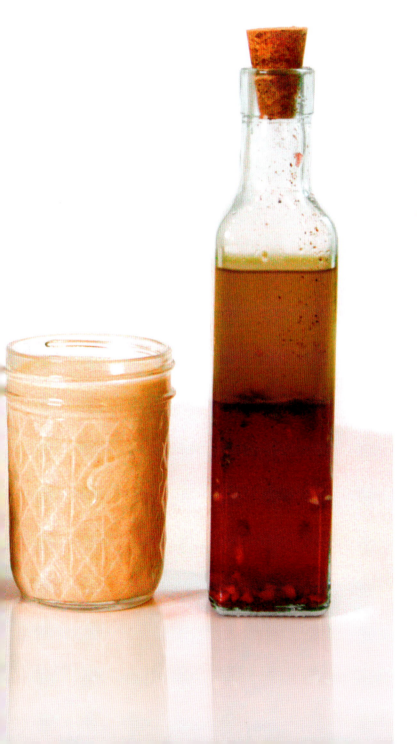

# 6
# DRIZZLE

## Dressings, Vinaigrettes + Sauces

It's always good to be saucy, especially when it's drizzled over your favorite dish. The right sauce elevates the presentation and essence of any fare. With our dressings, sauces, and spreads, there is never an excuse for a dull, dry meal. From fruity to spicy and savory to sweet, our Eat Fit Drizzles are culinary game changers.

# Oils 101

Low-fat is so 1980s. Essential fats are, well, essential for a healthy heart, brain, joints, and weight. But we get it: with so many oils to choose from, narrowing down the best options for cooking can be daunting. These are the 4 oils that cover most of our everyday culinary needs.

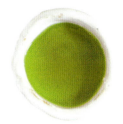

**AVOCADO OIL**  Rich in heart-smart fats with 70% monounsaturated fats.

**FLAVOR**  Slightly fruity with a very mild avocado flavor.

**HOW TO USE IT**  With a high smoke point, it's great for stir-frying, grilling, and sautéing. Its pretty green hue makes it a great choice for drizzling or dipping.

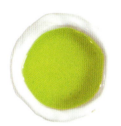

**EXTRA VIRGIN OLIVE OIL**  High in monounsaturated fats and rich in polyphenols, anti-inflammatories that help protect our body's cells from oxidative stress.

**FLAVOR**  The boldest, richest flavor of all types of olive oil.

**HOW TO USE IT**  With a low smoke point, it's best used for drizzling and dipping.

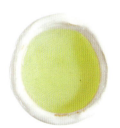

**EXTRA LIGHT OLIVE OIL**  Rich in heart-smart fats with 70% monounsaturated fats.

**FLAVOR**  No significant flavor profile.

**HOW TO USE IT**  With a relatively high smoke point, extra light olive oil is your new all-purpose cooking oil, taking the place of omega-6 rich vegetable oils.

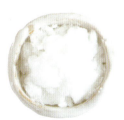

**COCONUT OIL**  Contains over 50% medium chain triglycerides (MCTs), which may be more easily burned as energy and less likely to be stored as fat.

**FLAVOR**  Coconut oil has a distinctly sweet, nutty flavor.

**HOW TO USE IT**  Solid at room temperature, coconut oil is an easy one-to-one substitute for butter.

# Miso Vinaigrette
*Chef Carl Schaubhut*

**Makes approximately ⅔ cup**

We also use this vinaigrette as a marinade for chicken and lean beef.

- 1 lime, zested and juiced
- 1 tablespoon rice vinegar
- ½ tablespoon minced garlic
- ½ tablespoon minced ginger
- 1 tablespoon minced shallot
- ½ tablespoon miso paste
- ⅓ cup light olive oil
- 1 teaspoon sesame oil

In a blender, blend 1 tablespoon lime juice with lime zest, vinegar, garlic, ginger, shallot, and miso. Slowly drizzle oils into blender. Blend well to emulsify.

**PER SERVING (2 TABLESPOONS):** 70 calories, 8 grams fat, 1 gram saturated fat, 35 mg sodium, <1 gram carbohydrate (<1 gram net carb), 0 fiber, 0 sugar, 0 protein

Low Carb, Vegan, Low Sodium

# Ginger Dressing
*Superior Grill*

**Makes approximately 1 cup**

Ginger lovers will want to make this simple drizzle over and over again.

- ½ cup water
- ¼ cup reduced sodium soy sauce
- 2 tablespoons Swerve Granular
- ½ cup pickled ginger
- ½ cup torn cilantro leaves

In a blender, combine all ingredients. Blend until smooth

**PER SERVING (2 TABLESPOONS):** 5 calories, 0 fat, 0 saturated fat, 210 mg sodium, 3 grams carbohydrate (1 gram net carb), 0 fiber, 0 sugar, 0 protein

Low Carb, Vegan

## Nutrition Bite /

Ginger helps to fight inflammation and improve digestion.

DRIZZLE

# Fresh Basil Vinaigrette
## Andrea's Restaurant

**Makes approximately ¾ cup**

This vividly hued vinaigrette will quickly become one of your go-to, everyday favorites.

- 1 tablespoon finely chopped white onion
- ½ teaspoon minced garlic
- 2 fresh basil leaves, chopped
- 1 teaspoon chopped fresh oregano
- ½ teaspoon sea salt
- ½ teaspoon freshly ground black pepper
- ⅔ cup extra virgin olive oil

Add all ingredients except olive oil to blender. Blend while slowly drizzling in olive oil to emulsify.

**PER SERVING (2 TABLESPOONS):** 200 calories, 24 grams fat, 3.5 grams saturated fat, 150 mg sodium, 0 carbohydrate (0 net carbs), 0 fiber, 0 sugar, 0 protein
**GF, Low Carb, Vegan**

# Cleo's Lemon Dressing
## Cleo's Mediterranean Cuisine & Grocery

**Makes approximately ⅔ cup**

Cleo's House Seasoning Blend adds layers of complexity to this simple vinaigrette.

- ¼ cup freshly squeezed lemon juice
- ¼ cup extra virgin olive oil
- 2 teaspoons white wine vinegar
- 2 teaspoons Cleo's House Seasoning Blend (page 91)

Add all ingredients except olive oil to blender. Blend while slowly drizzling in olive oil to emulsify.

**PER SERVING (2 TABLESPOONS):** 260 calories, 27 grams fat, 4 grams saturated fat, 250 mg sodium, 4 grams carbohydrate (4 grams net carbs), <1 gram fiber, <1 gram sugar (0 added sugar), 0 protein
**GF, Low Carb, Vegan**

# Tahini

**Makes 3 cups**

Nutty, creamy, and mild, this tahini sauce is a versatile addition to any dip, spread, or drizzle.

¼ cup lemon juice
2 cloves garlic, crushed
1½ cups raw tahini
1 teaspoon kosher salt
1¼ cups ice water, plus more as needed

Combine lemon juice and garlic in a nonreactive bowl; set aside for 30 minutes to steep.

Meanwhile, whip tahini in a stand or electric mixer on high speed for about 10 minutes, until it's glossy and light, like cake batter. It's nearly impossible to overwhip it, so feel free to spend a little time here.

Using a fine mesh strainer, separate the garlic from the lemon juice. Decrease the mixer's speed to medium and add garlic-infused lemon juice and salt. The tahini will seize up at first, but don't panic—just keep whipping it at medium speed and it will all come together.

When the tahini has a uniformly tacky, almost fudgy consistency, add ice water—about ¼ cup at a time—and increase the speed to high. The sauce may start to look almost curdled, but keep adding the ice water, whipping well after each addition. It will smooth out—the texture should be like that of a thick mousse. And know that every tahini is different. If, after you added all the water, it's still too thick, keep adding water by the tablespoon until it lightens up.

Prepared tahini will stay good for about 5-7 days in the fridge. If you're making it in advance, let it warm up just slightly on the counter, and whip in 1 to 2 tablespoons of ice water to restore some of its lightness.

**PER SERVING (2 TABLESPOONS):** 80 calories, 7 grams fat, 1 gram saturated fat, 80 mg sodium, 3 grams carbohydrate (3 grams net carbs), <1 gram fiber, 0 sugar, 2 grams protein
GF, Low Carb, Vegan, Low Sodium

# Labneh

**Makes 2-3 cups**

Creating the rich creaminess of labneh is fairly straightforward, despite taking time and planning. If you're pressed for time, go ahead and use full-fat, whole milk Greek yogurt instead.

**8 cups Bulgarian or Greek-style yogurt**
**1½ teaspoons kosher salt**

Fold a large 30-inch square of cheesecloth into eight layers and place it in a large sieve set over a deep nonreactive bowl.

In a separate bowl, combine yogurt with kosher salt, mix well. Pour into cheesecloth and cover the top loosely with plastic wrap. Allow to sit at room temperature overnight, giving the yogurt plenty of time to release all excess water.

After 12 to 15 hours, you should have 2 to 3 cups of thick, creamy labneh remaining in the cheesecloth, with the rest of the liquid in the bowl below. Using a spatula, scrape labneh into a container. Keep at room temperature to serve; otherwise store in an airtight container and refrigerate.

PER SERVING (2 TABLESPOONS): 30 calories, 1.5 grams fat, 1 gram saturated fat, 140 mg sodium, 1 gram carbohydrate (1 gram net carbs), 0 fiber, <1 gram sugar, 3 grams protein
GF, Low Carb, Vegetarian, Low Sodium

# Muhammara
*Saba*

**Makes 3 cups**

What originally landed in this book as a part of Saba's Charred Cabbage dish, this versatile smoky, savory, sweet, and spicy sauce is great for sandwiches, veggies, beef, chicken, or fish.

**1 batch Matbucha (recipe follows)**
**1¼ cups hazelnuts, toasted**
**3 tablespoons Aleppo pepper**
**1 teaspoon pomegranate molasses**
**¾ cup extra-virgin olive oil**

Combine Matbucha, hazelnuts, Aleppo pepper, and pomegranate molasses in food processor until nuts are finely chopped (you may need to pause and stir once or twice to keep everything moving).

While still blending, stream in olive oil and process until smooth. Allow to come to room temperature before serving. Refrigerate for up to four days, or freeze (tip: freeze in airtight containers the portions you plan to thaw and use).

## MATBUCHA

### Makes 2 cups

- 3 red bell peppers
- 5 tablespoons extra virgin olive oil, divided
- ½ yellow onion, thinly sliced
- 1 clove garlic, thinly sliced
- ½ teaspoon kosher salt
- 1½ teaspoons Aleppo pepper
- ½ teaspoon smoked paprika
- ½ teaspoon ground coriander
- ¼ teaspoon ground cumin
- 3 tablespoons white wine vinegar
- 1 15-ounce can peeled whole tomatoes
- 1½ teaspoons sugar

Broil peppers, or roast on a grill over a high flame, flipping midway thorough, until completely blackened with bits of papery white char, approximately 10-15 minutes, longer if needed.

After peppers have cooled, peel away charred skin (it can be helpful to keep your fingers wet as you do this, but don't run the peppers directly under the tap or you'll lose some smoky flavor). Remove the stem, seeds, and any remaining white pith or membrane. Roughly chop peppers and set aside.

Heat 2 tablespoons extra virgin olive oil in a wide, high-sided pan or Dutch oven over medium-low heat. Add onion and garlic, stirring occasionally until translucent but not brown, about 5 to 6 minutes.

Add salt, Aleppo pepper, smoked paprika, coriander, and cumin. Stir continually while ingredients toast and become fragrant. Add vinegar, stirring occasionally. All liquid should thicken.

Reduce heat to low. Add tomatoes, sugar, and red peppers. Use a spoon to break tomatoes apart roughly. Simmer gently. With the heat low enough that there's barely any movement in the pan, stir every so often to break up vegetables as they keep softening. After 1 to 1½ hours, when the matbucha is thick and dry with super concentrated flavors, remove from heat and stir in 3 tablespoons extra virgin olive oil. Cool completely before blending into muhammara.

**PER SERVING (2 TABLESPOONS):** 70 calories, 7 grams fat, 1 gram saturated fat, 35 mg sodium, 2 grams carbohydrate (2 grams net carbs), <1 gram fiber, 1 gram sugar (0 added sugar), <1 gram protein
GF, Low Carb, Vegan, Low Sodium

# Thai Peanut Dressing
## Blue Line Sandwich Co.

**Makes approximately 1 cup**

You'll want to make extra of this spicy and flavorful dressing because you'll be tempted to eat this with a spoon.

- ¾ cup creamy peanut butter
- 2 tablespoons seasoned rice vinegar
- ½ tablespoon reduced sodium soy sauce
- 1½ tablespoons honey
- ¾ teaspoon grated fresh ginger
- ½ tablespoon Sambal chili paste
- 2 tablespoons water

Whisk together peanut butter, vinegar, soy sauce, honey, ginger, and chili paste until well blended. Add water until dressing reaches desired consistency: pourable but still pretty thick.

**PER SERVING (2 TABLESPOONS):** 120 calories, 10 grams fat, 1.5 grams saturated fat, 150 mg sodium, 6 grams carbohydrate (5 grams net carbs), 1 gram fiber, 4 grams sugar (2 grams added sugar), 4 grams protein

LOW CARB, VEGETARIAN

## Ingredient Improv

Almond butter can be used in place of peanut butter. If you prefer to go entirely nut-free, use sunflower seed butter.

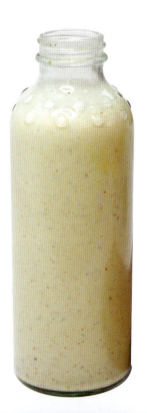

# Creole Lemon Vinaigrette
## Broussard's Restaurant

**Makes just under 1 cup**

We love that this refreshing—and pretty—vinaigrette is light, citrusy, and creamy.

- 2 lemons, zested and juiced
- 1 tablespoon Creole mustard
- 1 tablespoon honey
- ¼ cup Steen's cane vinegar
- ½ cup extra virgin olive oil
- 1 pinch sea salt
- 1 pinch freshly ground black pepper

Whisk together lemon zest, juice, mustard, honey, and vinegar. Slowly whisk in olive oil and season with salt and pepper.

**PER SERVING (2 TABLESPOONS):** 90 calories, 10 grams fat, 1.5 grams saturated fat, 50 mg sodium, 2 grams carbohydrate (2 grams net carbs), 0 fiber, 2 grams sugar (2 grams added sugar), 0 protein

GF, LOW CARB, VEGETARIAN, LOW SODIUM

# Raspberry Mint Vinaigrette
## Caffe! Caffe!

**Makes approximately 1 cup**

Caffe! Caffe! is well known for its impressive list of skillfully crafted homemade dressings, including this Raspberry Mint Vinaigrette. The sugar in the original version was a bit high for Eat Fit, so they dialed back the honey and added a touch of Swerve. And nobody complained. In fact, they're still asking for extra!

½ cup raspberry blush vinegar
½ tablespoon honey
1 tablespoon chopped fresh mint
½ teaspoon Swerve Granular
½ cup extra virgin olive oil

Add all ingredients except olive oil to blender. Blend while slowly drizzling in olive oil to emulsify.

**PER SERVING (2 TABLESPOONS):** 90 calories, 9 grams fat, 1 gram saturated fat, 0 sodium, 4 grams carbohydrate (4 grams net carbs), 0 fiber, 3 grams sugar (<1 gram added sugar), 0 protein

GF, Low Carb, Vegetarian, Low Sodium

# Poppyseed Berry Vinaigrette
## Dakota Restaurant

**Makes approximately 1½ cups**

Sweet, tart, and just a bit spicy, this vinaigrette is a fun addition to any fresh salad.

½ cup raspberry vinegar or raspberry blush vinegar
2 tablespoons Swerve Granular
½ cup julienned red onions
1 teaspoon dry mustard
2 teaspoons poppy seeds
1 teaspoon freshly ground black pepper
1 cup light olive oil

In a small skillet over medium heat, combine vinegar and Swerve and heat until mixture just reaches a simmer. Remove from heat, add red onions, and stir gently to soften. Allow to cool slightly. Stir in dry mustard, poppy seeds, and black pepper. Slowly add oil and whisk to blend.

**PER SERVING (2 TABLESPOONS):** 130 calories, 15 grams fat, 2 grams saturated fat, 0 sodium, 3 grams carbohydrate (1.5 grams net carbs), 0 fiber, <1 gram sugar (0 added sugar), 0 protein

GF, Low Carb, Vegan, Low Sodium

## Ingredient Improv

Champagne vinegar can be used in place of raspberry blush vinegar.

# Tea-Infused Berry Vinaigrette
## English Tea Room

**Makes nearly 2 cups**

Any low-sugar berry vinaigrette will work beautifully in this recipe. We prefer Hanley's because it's locally made and low in added sugar, with a simple, straightforward ingredient list.

**2 ounces freshly brewed raspberry tea**
**1 12-ounce bottle Hanley's Strawberry Vinaigrette**

Steep tea and allow to cool. In a large bottle or mason jar with an airtight lid, combine two ounces of tea and bottle of vinaigrette and shake well. Store refrigerated for up to 4 weeks.

**PER SERVING (2 TABLESPOONS):** 20 calories, 1.5 grams fat, 0 saturated fat, 95 mg sodium, 3 grams carbohydrate (3 grams net carbs), 0 fiber, 3 grams sugar (3 grams added sugar), 0 protein
GF, Low Carb, Vegan, Low Sodium

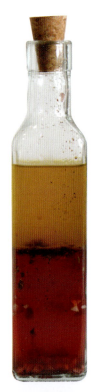

# Red Wine Vinaigrette
## Kingfish

**Makes approximately 1 cup**

If you're looking for a simple, traditional red wine and olive oil vinaigrette, this is right up your alley.

½ cup red wine vinegar
1 clove garlic, minced
1 teaspoon dried oregano
⅛ teaspoon sea salt
⅛ teaspoon freshly ground black pepper
½ cup extra virgin olive oil

In a blender, combine all ingredients. Blend until smooth.

**PER SERVING (2 TABLESPOONS):** 110 calories, 13 grams fat, 2 grams saturated fat, 30 mg sodium, 0 carbohydrate (0 net carbs), 0 fiber, 0 sugar, 0 protein
GF, Low Carb, Vegan, Low Sodium

# Steen's Cane Vinaigrette
## Commander's Palace

**Makes approximately 1 cup**

If Steen's Cane Vinegar isn't available, apple cider vinegar can be a good substitution. Of course, it's not the same, says Chef Meg, but it will do in a pinch.

- 1 clove garlic, minced
- ¼ cup apple cider vinegar
- ½ cup Steen's Cane Vinegar
- 2 tablespoons Lea & Perrins Worcestershire sauce
- 1 tablespoons Crystal hot sauce
- ½ teaspoon ground black pepper
- 1 teaspoon kosher salt
- ¼ cup extra virgin olive oil

Place all ingredients except oil in stainless steel bowl and whisk to combine. Slowly drizzle in oil. Season with additional salt and black pepper if needed.

**PER SERVING (2 TABLESPOONS):** 50 calories, 5 grams fat, 0.5 gram saturated fat, 270 mg sodium, <1 gram carbohydrate, 0 fiber, <1 gram sugar (0 added sugar), 0 protein
**GF, Low Carb, Vegan**

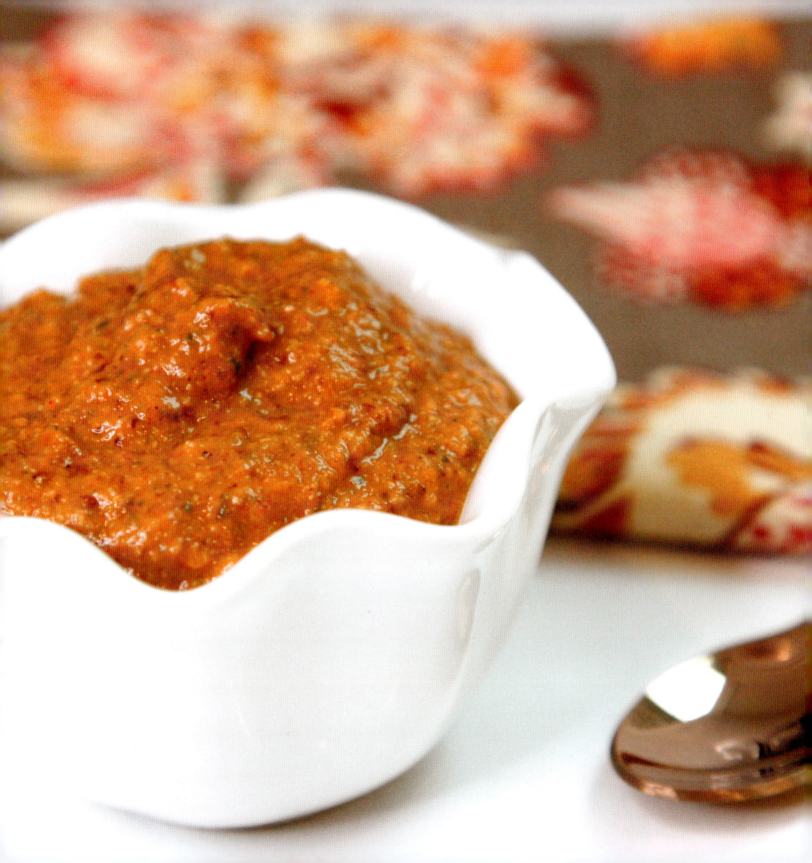

# Remoulade Sauce
## Galatoire's

**Makes approximately 4 cups**

Zingy and bold in flavor, this famous remoulade sauce is fabulous drizzled over anything and everything.

- ¾ cup chopped celery
- ¾ cup chopped scallions (white and green parts)
- ½ cup chopped curly parsley
- 1 cup chopped yellow onion
- ½ cup ketchup
- ½ cup tomato puree
- 2 tablespoons horseradish
- ½ cup Creole mustard or any coarse-grained brown mustard
- ¼ cup red wine vinegar
- 2 tablespoons Spanish hot paprika
- 1 teaspoon Lea & Perrins Worcestershire sauce
- ½ cup light olive oil

Mince celery, scallions, parsley, and onion in a food processor. Add ketchup, tomato puree, horseradish, mustard, vinegar, paprika, and Worcestershire sauce. Begin processing again, adding the oil in a slow drizzle to emulsify. Continue processing until dressing has reached a smooth consistency. Before serving, chill 6-8 hours or overnight.

**PER SERVING (2 TABLESPOONS):** 45 calories, 3 grams fat, 0 saturated fat, 110 mg sodium, 2 grams carbohydrate (2 grams net carbs), 0 fiber, 1 gram sugar (1 gram added sugar), 0 protein

GF, Low Carb, Low Sodium

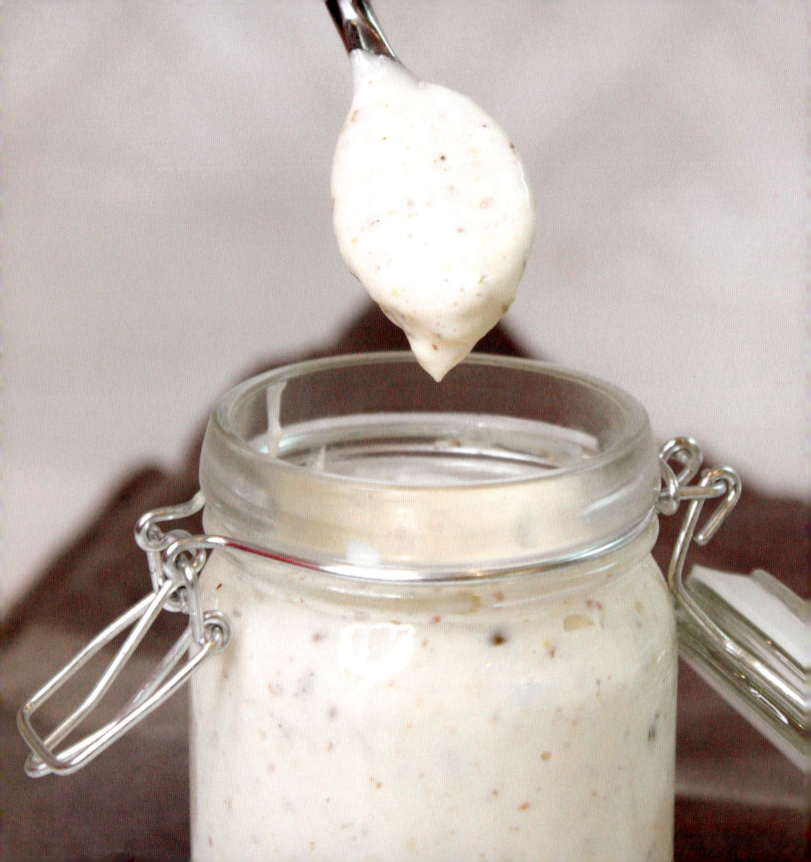

# Ravigote Sauce
## Eat Fit Collection

**Makes approximately 2¼ cups**

Tangy, creamy, and absolutely divine.

2 cups mayonnaise
1 tablespoon chopped capers
2 tablespoons horseradish
1 lemon, juiced
1 tablespoon Creole mustard
½ teaspoon hot sauce
¼ teaspoon Lea & Perrins Worcestershire sauce
1 tablespoon finely chopped onion
1 pinch sea salt
1 pinch freshly ground black pepper

In a large mixing bowl, combine all ingredients and stir until well combined.

**PER SERVING (2 TABLESPOONS):** 160 calories, 17 grams fat, 2.5 grams saturated fat, 190 mg sodium, <1 gram carbohydrate (<1 gram net carbs), 0 fiber, 0 sugar, 0 protein
**GF, LOW CARB**

## Nutrition Bite

Don't dis the mayo! Made simply of oil, egg yolks, and vinegar, this kitchen staple is naturally low in sodium and saturated fat. While calories can add up quickly, adding merely a drizzle of a mayonnaise-based cream sauce is an easy way to dial up texture and richness without breaking the nutritional bank.

## Love It Later

Refrigerate leftover ravigote for up to 4 days to dress up lean meats, fish, veggies, or just about anything.

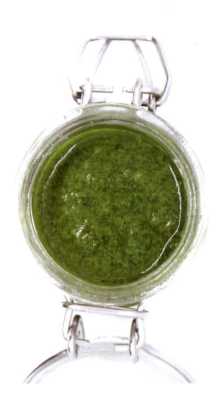

# Chimichurri
## *Parish Restaurant*

**Makes approximately 1½ cups**

This vibrant, zesty chimichurri bursts with flavors of fresh garlic, jalapeño, and lime.

½ cup parsley, finely chopped
½ cup cilantro, finely chopped
2 tablespoon shallots, finely chopped
1 fresh jalapeño, finely chopped (seeds removed for milder sauce)
2 cloves garlic, freshly grated
Half a lime, juiced
1 teaspoon red wine vinegar
1 teaspoon fish sauce
½ teaspoon dried oregano
¼ teaspoon dried Aleppo pepper
¾ cup extra virgin olive oil

Combine all ingredients in a container and add enough oil to cover.

**PER SERVING (2 TABLESPOONS):** 130 calories, 15 grams fat, 2 grams saturated fat, 45 mg sodium, 1 gram carbohydrate (1 gram net carbs), 0 fiber, 0 sugar, 0 protein
**GF, Low Carb, Low Sodium**

## By the Way /

We love Greek yogurt and use it often. We almost always recommend low fat (2%) plain Greek yogurt, never the fat free version. In fact, we really, really, really don't like fat-free Greek. It simply does not have the same texture, flavor, or richness as the low fat or full fat varieties. If you choose to go the nonfat route, don't say we didn't warn you.

# Chipotle Crema
## *Chef Carl Schaubhut*

**Makes approximately 2 cups**

This spicy-yet-cool sauce is one of our household staples; we love it with fish, steak, and vegetables, as well as with Chef Carl's Shrimp + Mirliton Stuffed Peppers (page 111).

1 cup 2% plain Greek yogurt
1 lime, zested and juiced
1 cup chipotle peppers in adobo sauce
½ teaspoon granulated garlic
¼ teaspoon sea salt

Blend together all ingredients. Refrigerate until ready to use.

**PER SERVING (2 TABLESPOONS):** 20 calories, 0 fat, 0 saturated fat, 190 mg sodium, 2 grams carbohydrate (2 grams net carbs), <1 gram fiber, 1 gram sugar (0 added sugar), 1 gram protein
**Low Carb, Vegetarian**

# Blueberry Beet Barbecue Sauce
## Commander's Palace

**Makes approximately 4 cups**

Fresh, local blueberries are our go-to for this sauce, but even outside of blueberry season you can whip up a batch with frozen blueberries.

- 3 medium red beets
- 2 tablespoons extra virgin olive oil
- 1 poblano pepper
- 2 cups blueberries, fresh or frozen
- ¼ cup coconut oil
- ½ cup yellow onion, diced
- 1 tablespoon ginger, finely chopped
- 2 tablespoons garlic, minced
- ¾ cup apple cider vinegar
- 3 tablespoons Swerve Brown Sugar Replacer
- 3 cups chicken stock
- 1 tablespoon kosher salt
- 2 tablespoons bourbon
- ½ teaspoon crushed red pepper flakes

Preheat oven to 350 degrees. Wash whole beets and place in roasting pan. Rub with olive oil and roast for 25-30 minutes or until soft enough to pierce with a fork. Let cool, then peel and chop, and set aside.

Increase oven temperature to 450 degrees. On an oiled baking sheet, roast poblano pepper and blueberries for 10 to 15 minutes, turning occasionally, until both berries and pepper are blistered. Set aside to cool.

Add coconut oil to a large saucepan over medium heat. Once sizzling, add onion, ginger, and garlic. Sauté until light golden brown, then add beets and sauté for an additional five minutes. Be sure to scrape the bottom of the pot with a wooden spoon to work all fond into vegetables.

Remove stem from cooled poblano and scrape pepper and berries into pot. Stir to combine. Add apple cider vinegar and Swerve Brown Sugar Replacer and again scrape to add all fond into sauce. Reduce by half and add chicken stock, salt, bourbon, and crushed red pepper flakes.

Bring to a simmer and adjust to low heat. Simmer for 60-90 minutes until beets are tender, then allow to cool before adding mixture to blender. Puree sauce to a velvet smooth consistency, then pass through a fine mesh sieve. If sauce seems too thin, add back to saucepan and simmer over low heat for another 20 minutes, until sauce reduces to desired consistency.

Store in the fridge for up to a week or freeze for up to three months.

**PER SERVING (2 TABLESPOONS):** 20 calories, 1.5 grams fat, 1 gram saturated fat, 100 mg sodium, 1 gram carbohydrate (1 gram net carbs), 0 fiber, <1 gram sugar (0 added sugar), 0 protein

GF, Low Carb, Low Sodium

# Mango Chutney
## FUEL Café + Market

**Makes 1½ cups**

Sweet, savory, and a little bit spicy, this chutney is the secret sauce—quite literally—for our Day-Brightening Curry Chicken Salad. It's also an easy way to take everyday favorites to the next level. Spread it onto sandwiches, serve it as a dipping sauce, or drizzle it over Greek yogurt, cottage cheese, or your favorite creamy cheese.

¼ cup liquid allulose
¼ cup unseasoned rice wine vinegar
½ teaspoon red pepper flakes
¼ teaspoon freshly ground black pepper
1 tablespoon curry powder
1½ teaspoon salt
½ cup unsweetened coconut flakes, lightly toasted
1 tablespoon grated fresh ginger
1 garlic clove, grated
1 ripe mango, grated (or ½ cup frozen mango cubes, thawed and chopped)
½ cup unsweetened canned coconut milk

Add all ingredients to a saucepan over high heat. Bring to a simmer for five minutes, stirring throughout. Remove from heat and allow the sauce to cool.

**PER SERVING (2 TABLESPOONS):** 30 calories, 2 grams fat, 1.5 grams saturated fat, 140 mg sodium, 3 grams carbohydrate (3 grams net carbs), <1 gram fiber, 2 grams sugar (0 added sugar), 0 protein

GF, Low Carb, Vegan, Low Sodium

# Eat Fit Berry Reduction
## The Eat Fit Collection

**Makes 1 cup**

This syrupy berry goodness was created for the low carb cheesecake in these pages. We also highly recommend adding a spoonful of this yumminess to Greek yogurt, cottage cheese, oatmeal, whole grain pancakes, or waffles; we promise you won't regret it.

1 cup frozen berries (blueberries, blackberries, and/or raspberries)
¼ cup water
¼ cup Swerve Granular
1 tablespoon lemon juice

Add berries, water, and Swerve to a medium saucepan over medium heat. Bring to a rolling boil, then reduce heat and simmer for 15-20 minutes. Remove from heat. Add lemon juice and whisk. Serve chilled or slightly warmed.

**PER SERVING (2 TABLESPOONS):** 5 calories, 0 fat, 0 saturated fat, 0 sodium, 2 grams carbohydrate (2 grams net carbs), 0 fiber, 1 gram sugar (0 added sugar), 0 protein

GF, Low Carb, Vegan, Low Sodium

# Maple Pecan Butter
## FUEL Café + Market

**Makes 1 cup**

Chef Ryan Conn of FUEL Café recommends a medium or larger food processor for nut butters, as a smaller blender may overheat the nuts and create a bitterness. It's a large mixing surface area, he says, that is one's friend when making nut butters.

**2 cups pecan halves or pieces**
**2 tablespoons Swerve Brown Sugar Replacer**
**¼ teaspoon sea salt**
**½ cup allulose syrup**

In an oven preheated to 350 degrees, bake pecans for 4-5 minutes, until lightly toasted. Once cooled, add toasted pecans, Swerve Brown Sugar Replacer, and sea salt into a medium food processor. Pulse 10 times or so to gently chop and mix ingredients together. Turn the food processor on and slowly drizzle in the allulose syrup. The pecan mixture may ball up like dough at first, but it will eventually smooth out into a spreadable paste after all the liquid has been added.

Refrigerate any extras in an airtight container for up to a week.

**PER SERVING (2 TABLESPOONS):** 110 calories, 12 grams fat, 1 gram saturated fat, 25 mg sodium, 2 grams carbohydrate (0 net carbs), 2 grams fiber, <1 gram sugar (0 added sugar), 1 gram protein
GF, Low Carb, Vegan, Low Sodium

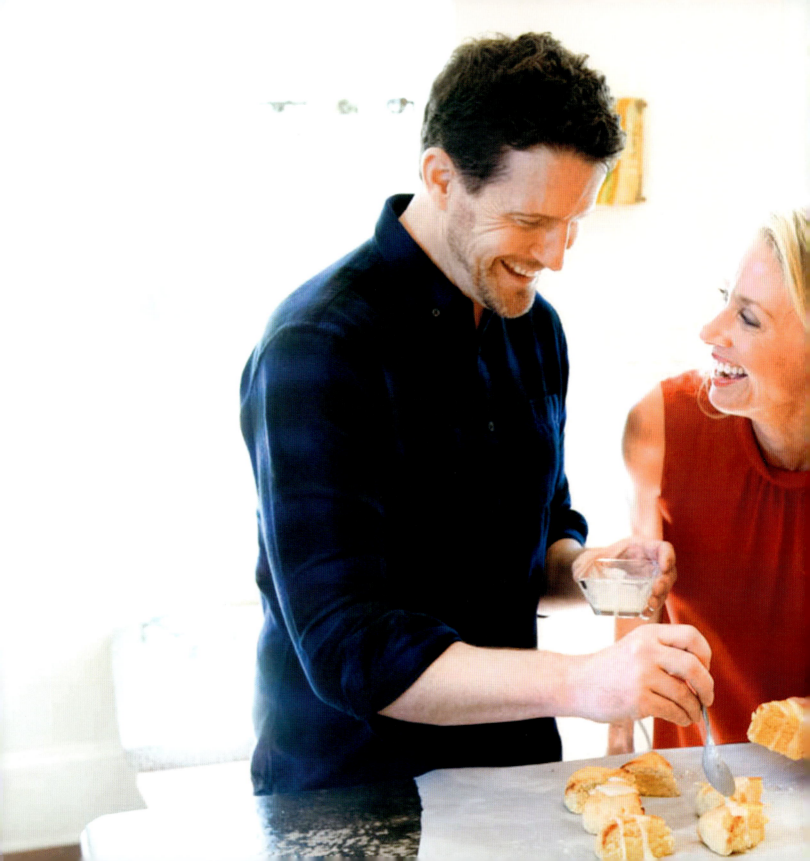

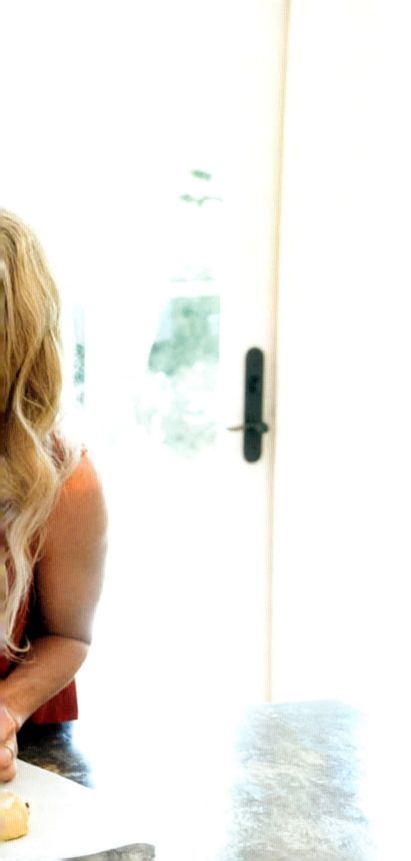

# 7
# INDULGE
## Sweets, Treats + Bakery

They said it was impossible! They said it couldn't be done! *Nothing* can tame the savage beast of the sweet tooth *and* help us stay on track with our health. Nothing, that is, until now.

Thanks to Eat Fit, it's now possible to treat yourself with our nutritious desserts that truly indulge the mind, body, and spirit. All of these sweet delights are gluten free, with little or no sugar added. You've got to try it to believe it!

# Swerve 101

Quite frankly, desserts are the biggest challenge for our Eat Fit restaurant partners. Fortunately, the selection of plant-based zero-calorie sweeteners continues to expand, making it easier than ever to dial back on added sugar, naturally.

As we were writing the original Eat Fit Cookbook, we turned to Swerve, our friend and partner in all things sweet, who has never met a dessert that they couldn't make effortlessly indulgent.

Swerve is a plant-based, all-natural, zero-calorie, non-glycemic sweetener that looks, measures, bakes, and sweetens just like sugar. This is important, because sugar doesn't just sweeten, it also browns and caramelizes while adding volume and moisture to our baked goods. Swerve does the same thing, sans the sugar.

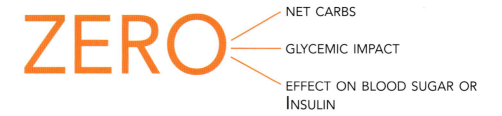

**CALCULATING NET CARBS**

Most carbs have 4 calories per gram. But plant-based sweeteners like erythritol and allulose change the "rules" about counting carbs, essentially providing ZERO calories per gram. Swerve is primarily erythritol, so when we use Swerve or pure allulose in a recipe, we subtract all of the carbs that they provide.

If you're using a recipe analysis program, simply subtract the grams of fiber and the grams of Swerve from the total carbohydrate count.

EXAMPLE A serving of our Rustic Eat Fit King Cake has 43 grams of total carbohydrates, 6 grams of fiber, and 32.5 grams of Swerve, resulting in 4.5 grams of net carbs per serving:

43 g CARBS – 6 g FIBER – 32.5g SWERVE = 4.5 NET CARBS per serving

# Swerve Sugar Replacement Options

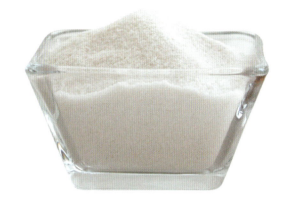

**SWERVE GRANULAR** White table sugar replacement; use it just like you would regular cane sugar.

**SWERVE CONFECTIONERS** Powdered sugar replacement; excellent for icing, frosting, pudding—anything where you need that smooth, silky texture.

**SWERVE BROWN SUGAR REPLACER** Brown sugar replacement; looks, smells, and tastes like brown sugar, providing molasses-type undertones of brown sugar.

**ALLULOSE** Available in granular or liquid form, allulose sweetens like sugar in a one-to-one ratio, like Swerve. It adds a bit more moisture to baked goods, and it works really well as a zero-calorie alternative to simple syrup.

## HIGH INTENSITY SWEETENERS

Natural sweeteners like Stevia and monkfruit are up to 200 times sweeter than sugar. While small amounts can work well in specific recipes, they can often be perceived as bitter—so you'll see that we don't include these in most recipes.

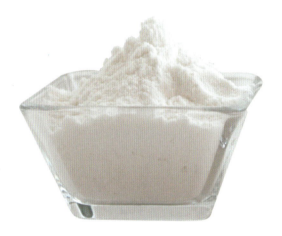

### Tips for Baking with Swerve

o   For frostings and icings or anytime a recipe calls for a lot of powdered sugar, cut the sugar in half when using Swerve Confectioners.

o   Cover baked goods with foil about halfway through baking so that the crust doesn't over-brown.

o   Keep Swerve sealed and stored in its original packaging or in an airtight resealable container to help it stay soft and pourable. It can also be refrigerated.

o   When baking with gluten-free flours, you'll typically need to add a small amount of xanthan gum, gelatin, or whey protein to provide the structure and texture of gluten.

Translation: If you remake a traditional recipe with gluten-free flour and wind up with a crumbly mess on your hands, add a touch of one of these gluten replacers to help tighten things up. Conveniently, several of the newer formulations of Swerve now already include xanthan gum.

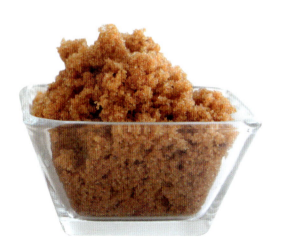

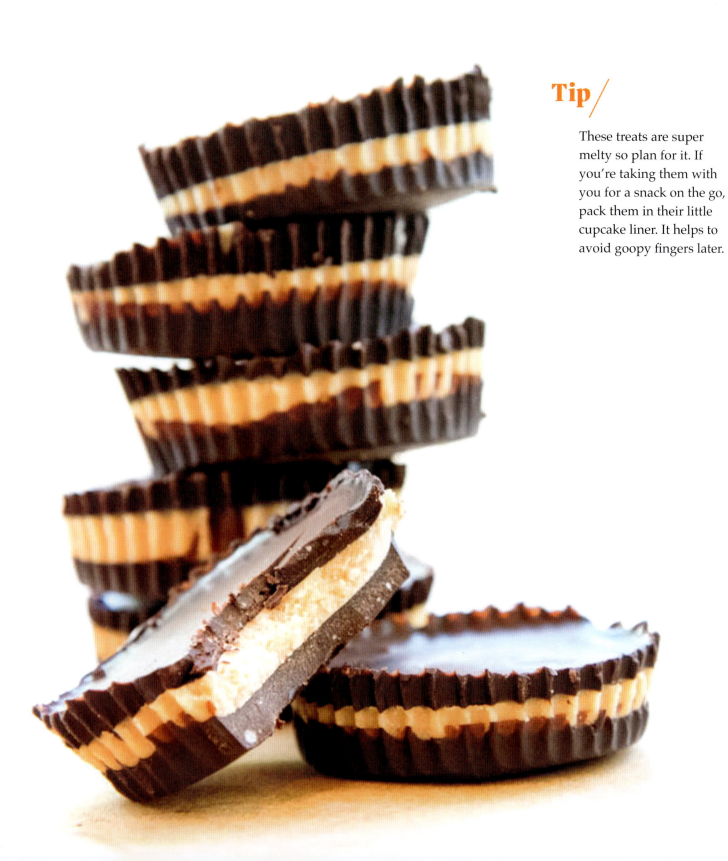

### Tip /

These treats are super melty so plan for it. If you're taking them with you for a snack on the go, pack them in their little cupcake liner. It helps to avoid goopy fingers later.

# Salted Dark Chocolate Peanut Butter Cups

*Eat Fit Collection*

**Makes 12 peanut butter cups**

We love peanut butter cups. Love-love-love them, like can't-keep-them-in-the-house love them. So we flipped over these low-carb versions that truly taste like the real thing.

**For the Chocolate Coating**
¾ cup coconut oil, melted
¾ cup unsweetened cocoa powder
¼ cup + 2 tablespoons Swerve Confectioners

**For the Peanut Butter Filling**
½ cup no-sugar-added creamy peanut butter
¼ cup cacao butter, melted
¼ cup Swerve Confectioners
1½ teaspoons sea salt

In a muffin pan, place liners into 12 cups. Set aside.

**Prepare the Chocolate Coating:** Whisk together melted coconut oil, cocoa powder, and Swerve in a medium bowl. Spoon 1 tablespoon of the chocolate mixture into each muffin liner. Freeze for 5 minutes or until mixture is no longer shiny on top.

**Make the Peanut Butter Filling:** Whisk together peanut butter, melted cacao butter, Swerve, and sea salt until combined. If it seizes up, microwave for 10 seconds.

Remove muffin pan from freezer and add 1 tablespoon of peanut butter mixture to the frozen chocolate coating. Return pan to freezer for 5-10 minutes.

After mixture has set, remove pan from freezer and add ½ tablespoon of the remaining chocolate mixture to each cup, covering the peanut butter layer. Freeze for 5-10 minutes until completely frozen. Store in fridge or freezer in an airtight container.

**PER SERVING (1 PEANUT BUTTER CUP):** 240 calories, 24 grams fat, 15 grams saturated fat (all plant-based), 240 mg sodium, 13 grams carbohydrate (2 grams net carbs), 3 grams fiber, <1 gram sugar (0 added sugar), 4 grams protein
GF, Low Carb, Vegan

## Ingredient Improv

These are equally decadent with almond butter, cashew butter, or sunflower seed butter.

## Note

Make ahead and store in the fridge or freezer. We like to let frozen cups soften for a few minutes first before eating.

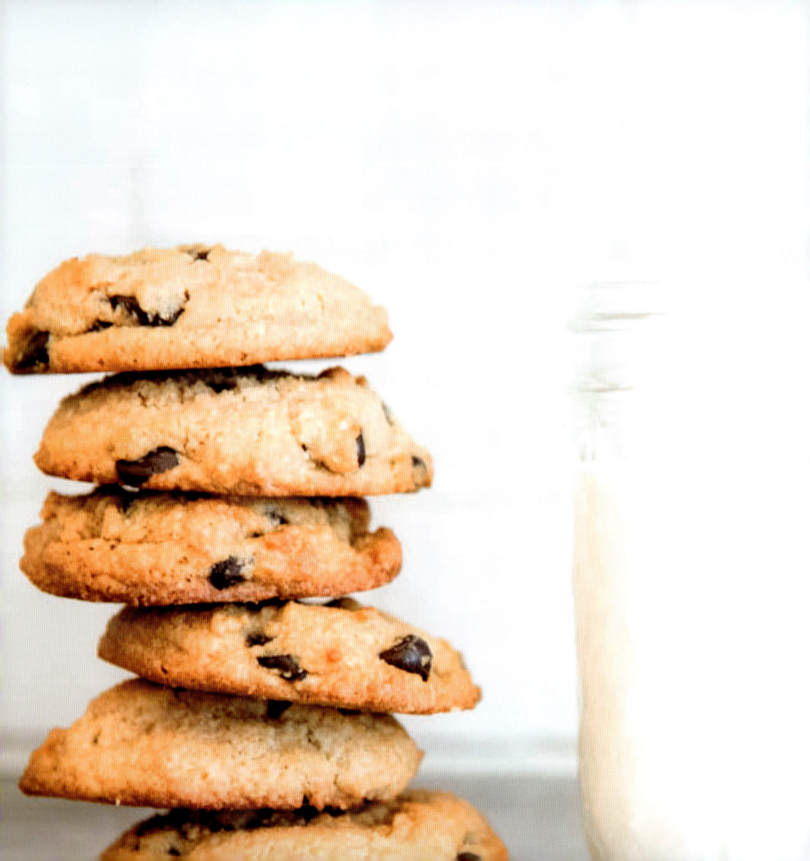

# Chocolate Chip Cookies
## Eat Fit Collection

**Makes 24 cookies**

Raise your hand if you love chocolate chip cookies! We do—especially when they are ooey-gooey soft on the inside and crispy-crunchy on the outside.

- 1½ cups almond flour
- 1 teaspoon powdered gelatin
- ½ teaspoon baking powder
- ½ teaspoon sea salt + extra for garnish
- ½ teaspoon baking soda
- 6 tablespoons unsalted butter (room temperature), divided
- ⅔ cup Swerve Brown Sugar Replacer
- 1 teaspoon vanilla
- 1 egg (room temperature)
- ⅛ cup unsweetened coconut milk or almond milk
- ½-1 cup dark chocolate or bitter sweet chips

Preheat oven to 350 degrees. Line 2 cookie sheets with parchment paper and set aside.

Mix together almond flour, gelatin, baking powder, salt, and baking soda in a medium bowl and set aside.

Melt 4 tablespoons butter in a saucepan over low heat. Pour into the bowl of a stand mixer. Add remaining 2 tablespoons room temperature butter to the melted butter. On medium speed, beat butter, Swerve Brown Sugar Replacer, and vanilla until creamy. Add egg and beat until combined. Gradually beat in flour mixture until combined. Stir milk into cookie dough until evenly mixed. Fold in chocolate chips.

Using a tablespoon to measure, scoop dough onto cookie sheet. Sprinkle each cookie with a dash of sea salt. Bake for 12-14 minutes. It's okay if the cookie looks undercooked in the middle. Remove from oven and allow the cookies to cool completely on the cookie sheet. The cookies will remain soft and gooey inside yet crunchy on the outside.

**PER SERVING (1 COOKIE):** 100 calories, 8 grams fat, 3 grams saturated fat, 180 mg sodium, 11 grams carbohydrate (3 grams net carbs), 1 gram fiber, 4 grams sugar (3 grams added sugar), 2 grams protein
GF, Low Carb

## Tip /

Take it even further and use sugar-free stevia-sweetened chocolate chips to cut back on added sugar.

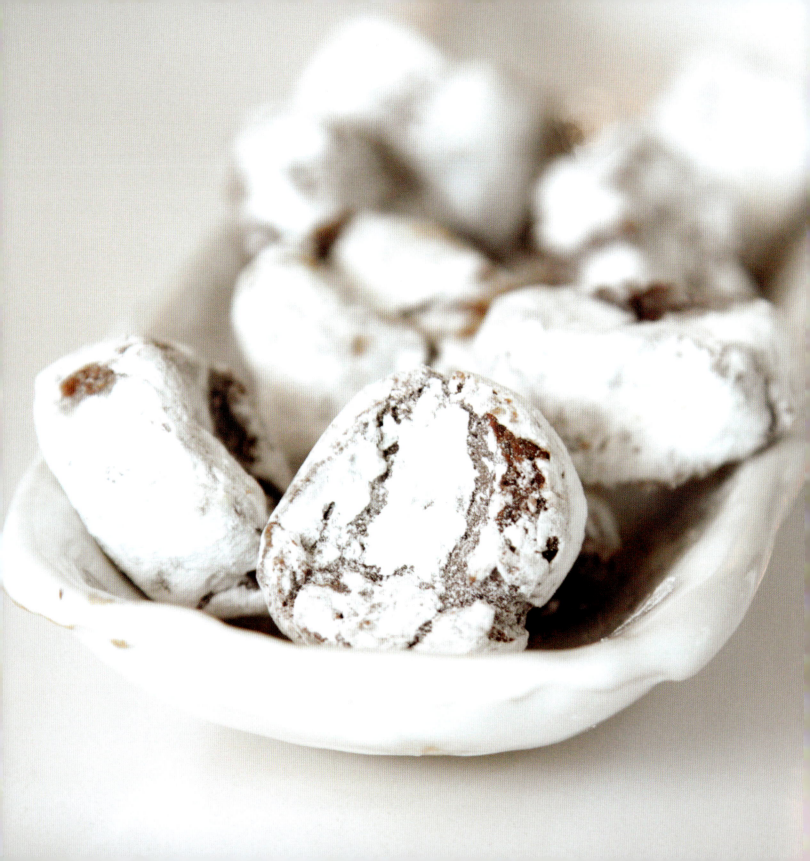

# Brutti Ma Buoni
## Eat Fit Collection

**Makes approximately 40 mini cookies**

If you've dined at Domenica in the Roosevelt New Orleans hotel, you probably remember the little bites of rich, chocolatey goodness that arrive in a little dish with the check. And no, they're not Eat Fit. But local artist (and Eat Fit advocate) Kristina Larson remade these decadent little treats with almond flour and Swerve, and we are beyond thrilled that they are just as good, if not even a little denser and richer.

- 2 tablespoons almond flour
- 1 tablespoon coconut flour
- ½ teaspoon baking powder
- ½ teaspoon salt
- 3 tablespoons unsweetened chocolate (100% cocoa), chopped
- ½ cup rounded, dark chocolate (at least 70% cocoa), chopped
- 2 tablespoons unsalted butter, softened
- 1 whole egg + 1 egg white (room temperature)
- ½ cup Swerve Granular
- 1 tablespoon finely ground espresso
- 1 teaspoons vanilla extract
- ½ cup stevia-sweetened semi-sweet chocolate chips (such as Lily's), frozen
- 2 tablespoons Swerve Confectioners, sifted

Sift flours, baking powder, and salt into a bowl and set aside.

Melt both varieties of unsweetened chocolate in a double boiler, taking care not to burn chocolate once it is melted. Whisk in butter.

In a separate bowl whisk together eggs and Swerve Granular until mixture becomes very thick and pale in color, approximately 6-8 minutes. Slowly stir in melted chocolate, occasionally scraping the sides of the bowl. Fold in flour mixture and scrape bowl again. Add espresso and vanilla extract and mix until combined. Do not overmix or the mixture will get too crumbly. Fold in frozen stevia-sweetened chocolate chips. Spread mixture onto a parchment-lined sheet pan. Cover lightly and refrigerate 12 hours or overnight.

Roll chilled mixture into balls about 1 inch in diameter. Press gently to flatten. Place cookies in freezer for at least 1 hour.

Preheat oven to 350 degrees. Roll batter in Swerve Confectioners, then arrange on a baking sheet. Bake for 10-12 minutes, until cookies are slightly puffed and fine lines or cracks appear. Remove from oven and transfer to parchment paper to cool. Sprinkle with additional Swerve Confectioners, if desired, before serving.

**PER SERVING (1 COOKIE):** 35 calories, 3 grams fat, 1.5 grams saturated fat, 40 mg sodium, 3 grams carbohydrate (2 grams net carbs), 1 gram fiber, <1 gram sugar (0 added sugar), <1 gram protein

GF, Low Carb, Vegetarian, Low Sodium

## By the Way

Brutti Ma Buoni is Italian for "ugly but good."

## Ingredient Note

Make sure to freeze the chocolate chips ahead of time. Otherwise they will melt while baking, and the cookies won't have chunks of chocolate.

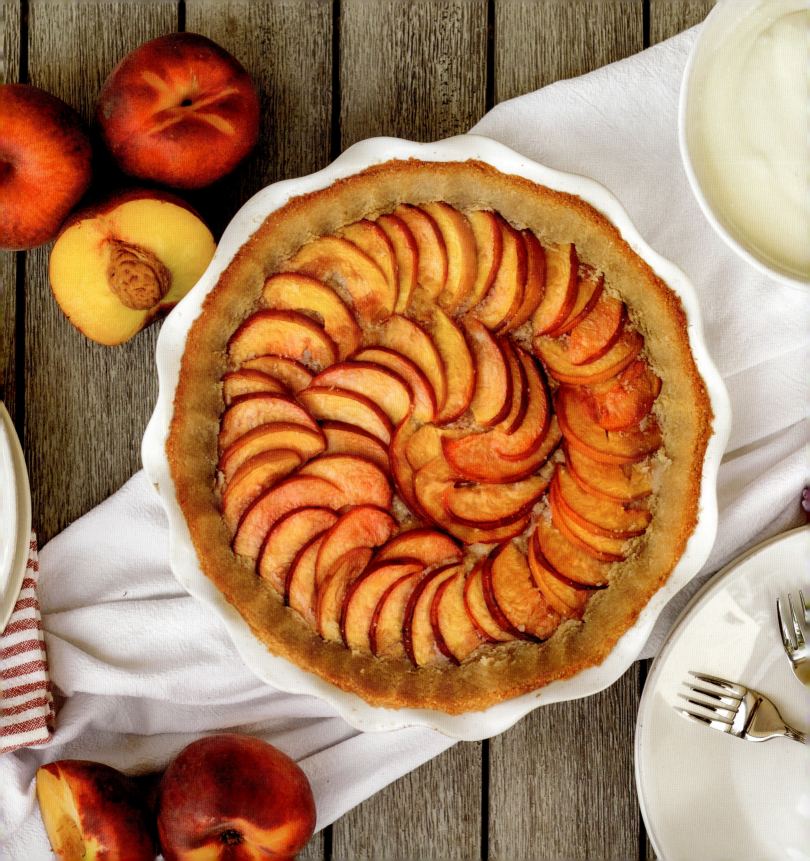

# Peach Pie with Whipped Goat Cheese
## Eat Fit Collection

**INDULGE**

**Makes 12 servings**

It's never a bad thing to carve out more time for homemade pie, especially when it's this good for you. Created by Ben McLauchlin, low carb baking aficionado and unofficial Eat Fit ambassador, you'll love this spin on classic peach pie that's naturally gluten free, with no added sugar.

### For the Crust
- 1¼ cups blanched almond flour
- ¼ cup coconut flour
- ¾ teaspoon xanthan gum
- ¼ cup Swerve Brown Sugar Replacer
- 3 tablespoons unsalted butter, melted
- 2-4 tablespoons cold water

### For the Filling:
- ½ cup Swerve Granular
- ¼ cup Swerve Brown Sugar Replacer
- 4½ cups sliced peeled peaches
- ¼ teaspoon ground nutmeg
- ¼ teaspoon ground cinnamon
- ⅛ teaspoon salt
- 2 teaspoons lemon juice
- 2 tablespoons butter
- 1 fresh peach

### For the Whipped Goat Cheese:
- 4 ounces goat cheese, room temperature
- 6 tablespoons heavy cream
- 1½ tablespoons Swerve Confectioners
- ¼ teaspoon pure vanilla extract

Preheat oven to 325 degrees. Grease a 9-inch pie pan and set aside. In a mixing bowl, combine all almond flour, coconut flour, xanthan gum, and Swerve Brown Sugar Replacer. Add butter, and with a fork, mix into dry ingredients until well-combined, with a cornmeal-like texture.

Gradually add water by the tablespoon until mixture sticks together but is not too wet or gummy.

Press dough evenly into pie pan. Bake for 10-12 minutes. Remove and let cool before adding filling.

In a large bowl, combine Swerve Granular and Swerve Brown Sugar Replacer. Add peeled peaches and toss gently to coat, then cover and let stand for 1 hour. Drain peaches in a colander placed over a bowl, reserving the juice.

In a small saucepan over medium heat, combine the nutmeg, cinnamon, and salt; gradually stir in reserved juice and bring to a boil. Stir for 2 minutes or until thickened. Stir in lemon juice and butter and whisk. Set aside for 7 minutes. Pour mixture over peaches in separate large mixing bowl and gently fold in. Pour into prepared pie crust.

Slice the fresh peach into thin slices and arrange over the top of the pie in a circular pattern.

While the peaches soak in the sweetener blend, prepare the Whipped Goat Cheese:

In a large bowl or stand mixer, mix the goat cheese, heavy cream, Swerve Confectioners, and vanilla on high speed for 5 minutes, scraping the sides as necessary. Cover and refrigerate until ready to serve.

Increase oven to 350 degrees and bake pie for 30 minutes, covered loosely with foil. After 30 minutes, remove foil and bake uncovered for another 10 minutes, until crust is golden brown and filling is bubbly. Remove from oven and cool on a wire rack. Serve warm or at room temperature, topped with a dollop of chilled Whipped Goat Cheese.

**PER SERVING:** 200 calories, 16 grams fat, 7 grams saturated fat, 80 mg sodium, 11 grams carbohydrate (7 grams net carbs), 3 grams fiber, 7 grams sugar (0 added sugar), 5 grams protein

**GF, LOW CARB, LOW SODIUM**

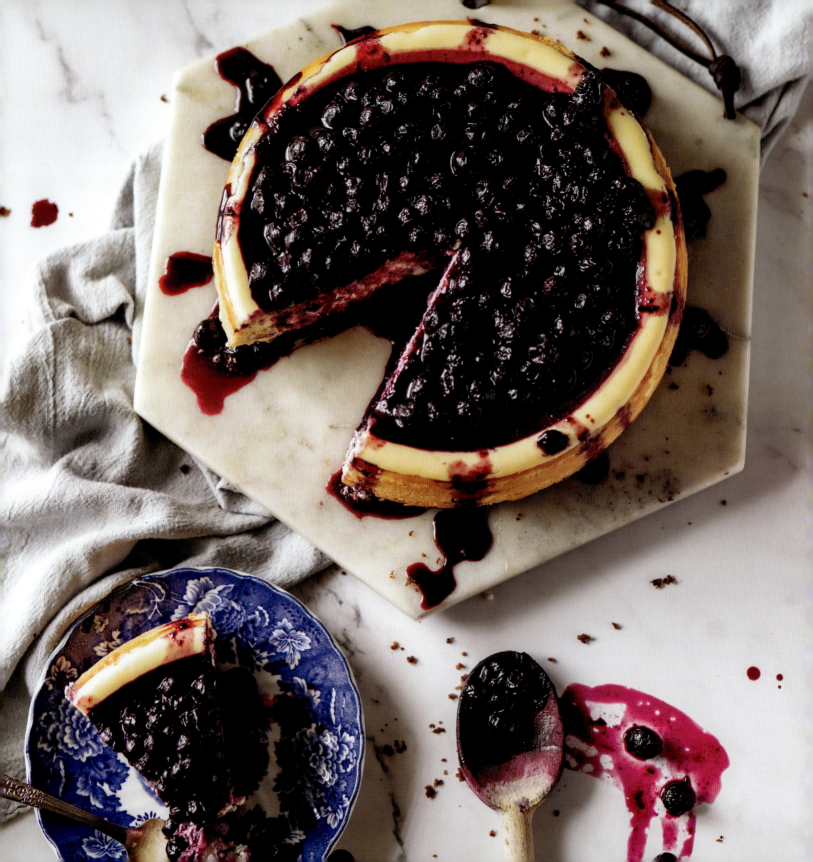

# Artisan Berry Cheesecake
## Caster and Chicory

**Makes 16 servings**

Richly decadent and stunningly low in carbs, this gorgeous cheesecake is also naturally gluten free. We love pairing it with our Eat Fit Berry Reduction; it's also brilliantly close to perfection with a drizzle of melted Lily's no-sugar chocolate chips (white, dark, or milk chocolate) or simply served solo.

**For the Crust**
1½ cups pecan flour or almond flour
¼ cup Swerve Granular
4 tablespoons butter, melted

**For the Filling**
24 ounces cream cheese, room temperature
1 cup Swerve Confectioners
3 eggs
½ cup sour cream
1½ teaspoons vanilla extract
⅛ teaspoon sea salt

**For the Topping (optional)**
1 batch of Eat Fit Berry Reduction (page 186)

Preheat oven to 325 degrees. In a medium mixing bowl, add pecan or almond flour, Swerve Granular, and butter. Mix until well-combined. Press into the bottom of a greased 10-inch springform pan. Refrigerate for 20 minutes.

Mix cream cheese and Swerve Confectioners with a mixer until light and fluffy. Add eggs, one at a time, beating on low speed, scraping sides as needed. Mix well. Add sour cream, vanilla, and sea salt. Mix until combined. Pour over the prepared crust.

It is important to bake this cheesecake slowly to reduce the chance of cracking (but don't worry if it does crack a bit, we sort of like the imperfections. Plus, the Berry Reduction helps to hide any flaws). Bake for 30 minutes, placing a baking sheet on the rack below to catch any run-off. Reduce oven temperature to 275 and continue baking for 45 minutes. After 45 minutes, turn off oven, leaving cheesecake inside for another 30 minutes. Be patient—don't open that door! After 30 minutes, crack the oven door just a bit to allow cheesecake to cool slowly for another hour.

Remove cheesecake from the oven and bring to room temperature on the counter, another 2-3 hours, then cover with plastic wrap and refrigerate. Serve chilled, topped with Eat Fit Berry Reduction.

**PER SERVING:** 260 calories, 23 grams fat, 11 grams saturated fat, 180 mg sodium, 8 grams carbohydrate (7 grams net carbs), 1 gram fiber, 3 grams sugar (0 added sugar), 7 grams protein
GF, Low Carb

## Love it Later

This cheesecake freezes fabulously. If sliced, wrap each piece tightly with plastic wrap. To freeze the entire cake, place it on a dish or cardboard round and cover snugly with plastic wrap.

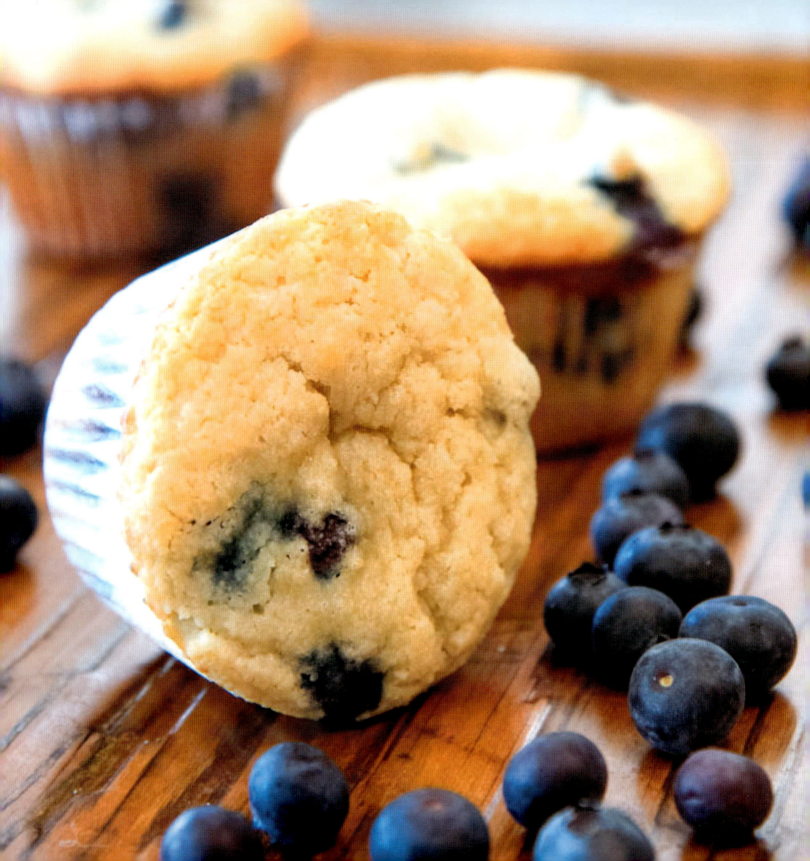

# Blueberry Protein Muffin
## Eat Fit Collection

**Makes 12 muffins**

It can be a challenge to get enough protein at breakfast—especially if we tend to reach for bread-heavy favorites like muffins and waffles. And too little protein, combined with too many carbs, can leave us feeling bottomed out in no time. But if you're craving a sweet treat for the first meal of the day, you're going to love these protein-rich, no-sugar-added muffins.

1½ cups finely ground almond flour
½ cup coconut flour
½ teaspoon sea salt
1 cup unsweetened protein powder
2 teaspoons baking powder
1 teaspoon baking soda
¼ cup melted butter
1 cup Swerve Granular
3 large eggs (room temperature)
¾ cup unsweetened almond milk
¼ cup 2% plain Greek yogurt
2 teaspoons lemon zest or ¼ teaspoon lemon extract
1 teaspoon vanilla extract
1½ cups fresh or frozen blueberries

**For the Topping (optional):**
3 tablespoons Swerve Granular
½ teaspoon ground cinnamon

Preheat oven to 325 degrees. Grease 12 wells of a standard muffin pan or line with muffin papers.

In a medium-sized bowl, stir together flours, salt, protein powder, baking powder, and baking soda; set aside. Whisk together the melted butter, Swerve, eggs, almond milk, yogurt, lemon zest or extract, and vanilla. Stir the dry mixture into the wet ingredients. Scrape the bottom and sides of the bowl and continue to mix just until blended (a few lumps will remain). Fold in the berries, then fill the muffin cups almost full. Top with Swerve mixed with ground cinnamon.

Bake for 15-20 minutes, until a toothpick inserted into the center of a muffin comes out clean. Remove the muffins from the oven and allow to rest for 5 minutes before transferring them to a rack to cool. These are also delicious served warm.

**PER SERVING (1 MUFFIN):** 200 calories, 13 grams fat, 4 grams saturated fat, 350 mg sodium, 25 grams carbohydrate (5.5 grams net carbs), 4 grams fiber, 3 grams sugar (0 added sugar), 12 grams protein
**GF, LOW CARB, VEGETARIAN**

## Fresh or Frozen?

When it comes to fruit, frozen is just as nutritious as fresh. Just check the ingredient list to be sure no sugar has been added. You can also stock up on fresh, seasonal berries when the price is right and freeze them for out-of-season use.

## Ingredient Improv

Trade out the blueberries for cranberries, blackberries, bananas, or whatever you have on hand. You really can't mess it up.

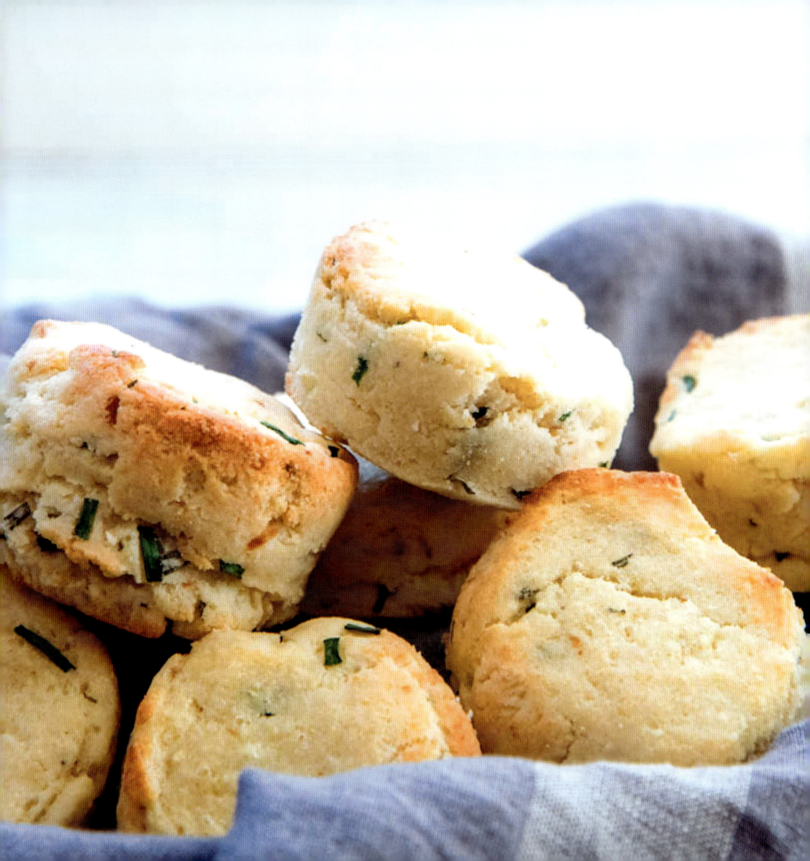

# Rosemary Garlic Biscuits
## *Eat Fit Collection*

**Makes 10 biscuits**

These savory little biscuits are fabulous on their own, perfect for brunch, and great at dinner as a fancier (and better for you) bread option.

- 1¾ cups almond flour
- ¼ cup coconut flour
- 2½ teaspoons baking powder
- ¼ teaspoon salt
- 4 tablespoons Swerve Granular
- 1 tablespoon chopped fresh rosemary
- 2 tablespoons chopped fresh chives
- ½ tablespoon chopped garlic
- 4 tablespoons coconut oil, chilled
- 1 egg (room temperature)
- 4 tablespoons unsweetened almond milk

Preheat oven to 350 degrees. Grease a baking sheet or round baking pan. In a medium-sized bowl, mix together almond and coconut flour with next 6 ingredients. Work coconut oil into flour mixture with a fork or your hands until it resembles breadcrumbs. Set aside.

In a small bowl beat together egg and milk. Add 5 tablespoons of the egg-milk mixture to the flour mixture (leaving a little egg and milk for basting the top of the biscuits) and mix until well combined.

Transfer dough to an almond-floured countertop or cutting board. Shape the dough into a circle about 2 inches thick. Using a buttered champagne flute or small biscuit cutter, cut biscuits out of dough. Place biscuits close together on a cookie sheet (when they cook you want the edges to touch so they stay soft). Bake for 15-20 minutes, or until tops are golden brown around the edges and the dough is cooked through. Remove biscuits from oven and transfer them to a bowl lined with a bread cloth, cloth napkin, or kitchen towel to keep the biscuits moist and warm for serving.

**PER SERVING (1 BISCUIT):** 220 calories, 18 grams fat, 8 grams saturated fat, 180 mg sodium, 14 grams carbohydrate (6 grams net carbs), 3 grams fiber, 2 grams sugar (0 added sugar), 7 grams protein

GF, Low Carb, Vegetarian

## Serve It Up

We love to make breakfast sandwiches out of these. My personal favorite is egg, goat cheese, and a slice of prosciutto.

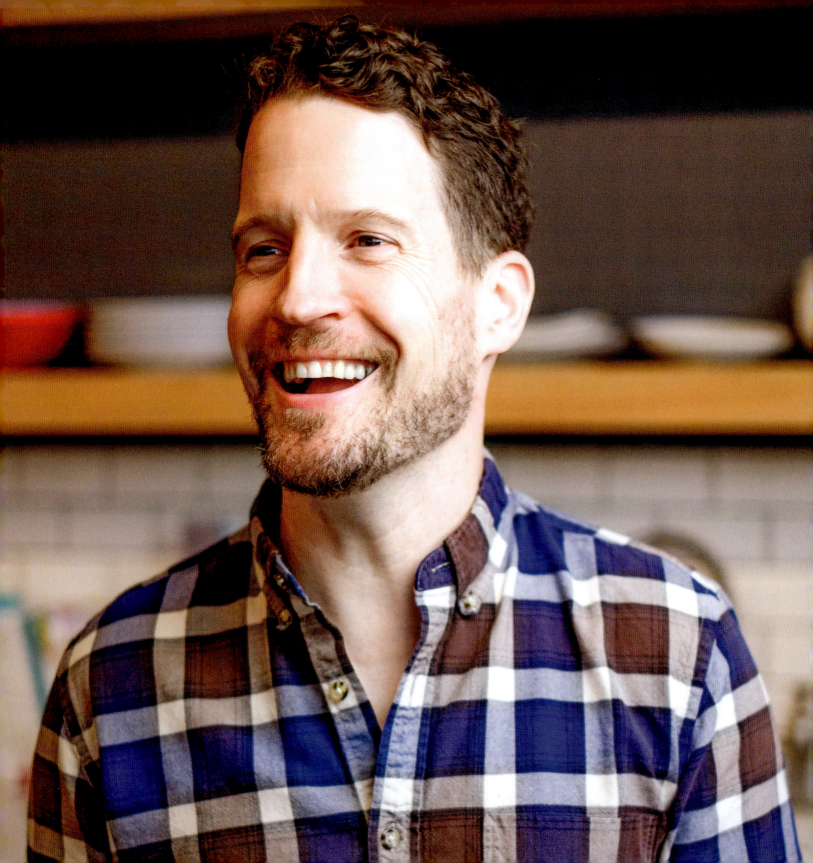

# Ben McLauchlin
## Low Carb Baking Aficionado

Ben is one of my favorite people on the planet. Compassionate and hilarious, he immediately dials in to the people around him to ensure that everyone is comfortable, happy, and, of course, well fed. I love collaborating and brainstorming with him on ideas and then watching (and tasting) as he creates nutritious deliciousness that exceeds all expectations.

For years, Ben served as the sales director for Swerve, but his unofficial title even now could be bakery R&D, as he's often in the kitchen re-working and re-creating traditional favorites into low-carb, low-sugar, gluten-free, and grain-free indulgences. And thanks to his incredible attention to detail, they're not only nutritious and delicious, they're visually stunning as well.

Back in the day, Ben baked Paula Deen-style: traditional Southern, with lots of white flour and sugar, sugar, sugar. But as wellness and nutrition have become a priority in his own life, his approach to baking has shifted: "I like to take my mom and my grandma's recipes, those that are part of my favorite memories as a kid, and re-make them to be low carb, grain-free, gluten-free, and no sugar added, essentially creating the sweets and treats that I want to eat but made with ingredients that align with how I prefer to fuel my body these days."

It's also important to Ben that others have the opportunity to experience and savor the decadent foods that we crave but made with good-for-you ingredients that we can feel good about. He takes any opportunity to expose friends and family to healthier options, serving lower-sugar desserts at tailgates, parties, and even his own wedding. And he always takes a quick minute to educate and inspire new fans to start making small changes on their own at home, encouraging them to "get their Swerve on."

> "I'm a country cook, y'all, and I love to bake. To me, food is love. And food immediately brings us back to our homes, our families, our memories, no matter where we are."
>
> —Ben McLauchlin

(Courtesy Mike Hartnett)

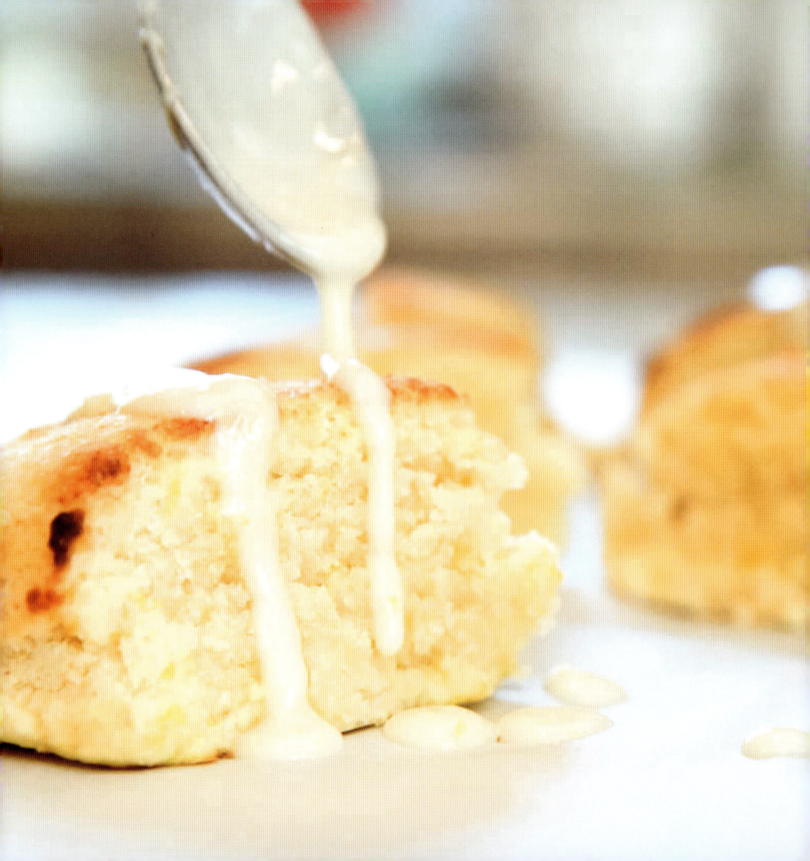

# Lemon Scones

## Eat Fit Collection

**Makes 8 scones**

Regardless of the season, it's immediately sunny and springtime with these lemon scones—perfect for brunch, a shower, or just an afternoon snack.

- 1¾ cups almond flour
- ¼ cup coconut flour
- 2½ teaspoons baking powder
- ¼ teaspoon salt
- 6 tablespoons Swerve Granular
- 2 tablespoons lemon zest
- 2 tablespoons unsalted butter, chilled
- 2 tablespoons coconut oil, chilled
- 1 egg (room temperature)
- 4 tablespoons unsweetened almond milk
- 1 teaspoon vanilla

### For the Glaze
- ¼ cup Swerve Confectioners
- 2 tablespoons fresh lemon juice
- ½-1 teaspoon lemon zest

Preheat oven to 350 degrees. Grease a baking sheet or round baking pan. In a medium-sized bowl, mix together dry ingredients and lemon zest. Grate butter into flour mixture (we like to use a cheese grater). Work coconut oil into flour mixture with a fork or your hands until it resembles breadcrumbs. Set aside.

In a small bowl, beat together egg and milk. Add 5 tablespoons of the egg-milk mixture to the flour mixture (leaving a little egg and milk for basting the top of the scones) and mix until well combined.

Transfer dough to parchment paper or an almond-floured countertop or cutting board. Shape the dough into a circle about 1½ inches thick. With a knife, cut the dough into 8 triangles. Place scones close together on a cookie sheet so that the edges of each scone just touch (when they cook you want the edges to touch so they stay soft). Bake for 15-20 minutes, or until tops are golden brown around the edges and the dough is cooked through. Remove from oven, set aside, and let cool.

**While Scones are cooling, prepare the Glaze:** In small bowl mix together Swerve Confectioners, lemon juice, and lemon zest until well combined. Sweeten to taste, as lemon can vary in tartness. Drizzle or brush onto cooled scones. Serve immediately. Store in an airtight container in fridge or freezer.

**PER SERVING (1 SCONE):** 230 calories, 20 grams fat, 6 grams saturated fat, 220 mg sodium, 23 grams carbohydrate (4 grams net carbs), 5 grams fiber, 2 grams sugar (0 added sugar), 7 grams protein

GF, Low Carb, Vegetarian

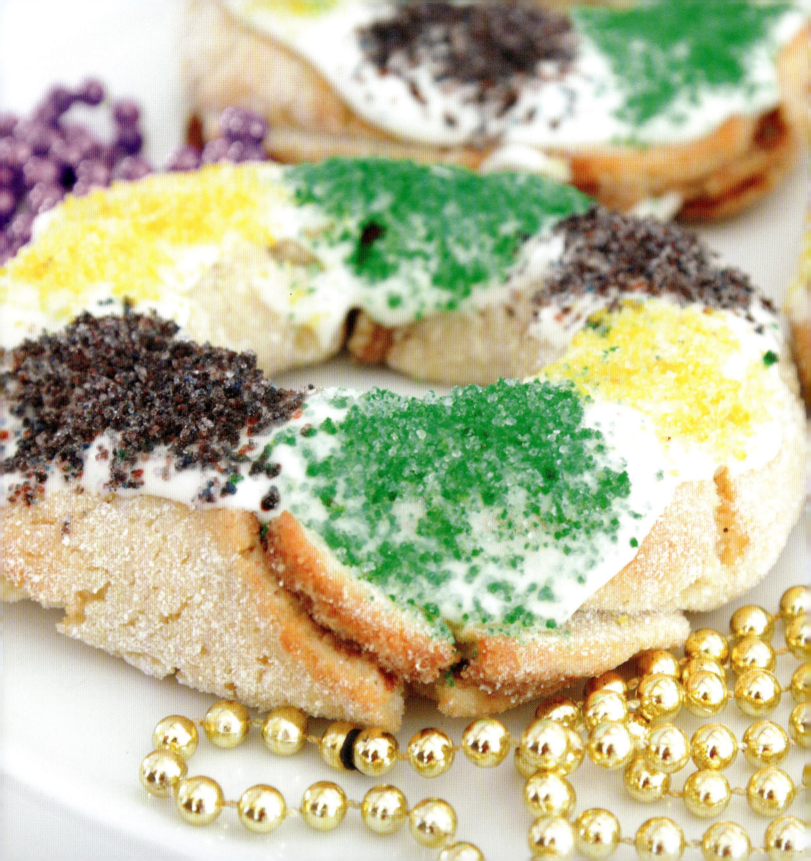

# Rustic Eat Fit King Cake
## Eat Fit Collection

**Makes 6 mini king cakes**

This king cake recipe by Ben McLauchlin was the inspiration for the Eat Fit king cake available in retail stores during Carnival season. I worked closely with Ben to scale up this recipe while still maintaining the specialty features that make it Eat Fit, not to mention keeping it gluten free, low carb, diabetic friendly, and keto approved.

**For the Cake**
- 2 cups fine almond flour
- 1 cup coconut flour
- ½ cup unsweetened protein powder
- 1 tablespoon baking powder
- 1 cup Swerve Granular
- 1 package unflavored gelatin
- ¼ cup sugar (to activate the yeast)
- 1 teaspoon sea salt
- 1 packet quick-rise yeast
- ½ cup whole milk (room temperature)
- ¼ cup water
- 6 tablespoons unsalted butter (room temperature), cut into tablespoons
- 3 eggs (room temperature)
- ¼ cup sour cream
- Butter for greasing pan and bowl

**For the Filling**
- ⅔ cup Swerve Granular
- 4 tablespoons ground cinnamon
- 8 ounces cream cheese, softened

**For the Glaze**
- 4 ounces cream cheese (room temperature)
- 2 tablespoons butter (room temperature)
- 6 tablespoons Swerve Confectioners
- 4 tablespoons milk
- 1 teaspoon vanilla

**For the Sprinkles**
- 1 cup Swerve Granular
- Natural food coloring (yellow, green, red, and blue)

In a medium bowl, whisk together almond flour, coconut flour, protein powder, baking powder, Swerve, and gelatin (we'll call this the flour mixture). Transfer 1½ cups of the flour mixture to a separate bowl. Using an electric mixer, combine the 1½ cups flour mixture with sugar, salt, and yeast (we'll call this the yeast mixture).

In a small saucepan over low heat, heat milk, water, and butter to 120-130 degrees. Stir into the yeast mixture and beat on medium until combined. Beat in eggs one at a time, then add sour cream and ½ cup of the flour mixture. Beat on medium-high until evenly mixed, approximately 1-2 minutes. Add the remaining flour mixture and continue beating an additional 1-2 minutes on medium-high to fully combine. Dough will be pliable and sticky.

Lightly butter a large mixing bowl. Shape dough into a ball and transfer to the mixing bowl, turning the dough to butter the surface on all sides. Cover bowl with a damp, warm, lightweight towel and place in a warm, draft-free area until the dough doubles in size, approximately 1 hour. Punch dough down, but do not overwork the dough. Cover with a warm, damp towel and set aside in a warm area to rise for another 30-60 minutes.

**Note**

If a warm, draft-free spot is not available, preheat oven to 150-175 degrees, turn off the oven, and crack the door to release some heat. Place the dough in the oven then close the oven door.

After allowing the dough to rise, divide dough in half and shape into 2 balls. (If the dough is too sticky to work with, refrigerate the dough for 10 minutes.)

Preheat oven to 350 degrees. Line 2 large baking sheets with parchment paper.

Lay out a separate large piece of parchment paper and lightly flour the rolling surface with coconut flour. Place one of the balls of dough onto the parchment paper and sprinkle with coconut flour. Lay a second sheet of parchment paper on top of dough, then roll out dough into a 12x12 inch square. Remove the top layer of parchment paper.

**Add the Filling:** Combine Swerve and cinnamon in a small bowl. Spread half of the softened cream cheese over the dough. Sprinkle half of the Swerve and cinnamon mixture on top.

Fold the dough by gently lifting one edge of the parchment paper, allowing the edge of the dough to roll over onto the cream cheese filling by about 2 inches. Repeat on the opposite side. Cover with parchment paper, and use the rolling pin to roll out the dough to its original 12x12 inch size.

With a pizza roller or knife, cut the dough into 3 equal strips. Transfer each strip to a baking sheet and shape each into an oval. Pinch the ends together using water-moistened fingers to seal. If the dough cracks when you create the oval, re-seal by pinching dough together.

Repeat process for the remaining ball of dough.

Bake for 17-20 minutes, or until cakes are lightly golden on top. Remove from oven and allow to cool for 30 minutes.

**While Cakes are baking, make the Glaze and the Sprinkles:** Beat together cream cheese and butter until smooth. Sift Swerve Confectioners into the mixture and whisk until creamy. Add milk and vanilla and whisk until combined. Set aside and make the sprinkles.

For the sprinkles, divide the granulated Swerve into 3 small bowls. Add natural yellow food coloring to one bowl and mix with a fork until the Swerve is completely yellow. Repeat with green and purple (equal parts red + blue) coloring.

Spread cream cheese glaze onto each cooled mini king cake and top with sprinkles.

**PER SERVING (¼ MINI KING CAKE):** 170 calories, 12 grams fat, 5 grams saturated fat, 160 mg sodium, 43 grams carbohydrate (5 grams net carbs), 6 grams fiber, 6 grams sugar (2 grams added sugar), 8 grams protein
**GF, LOW CARB**

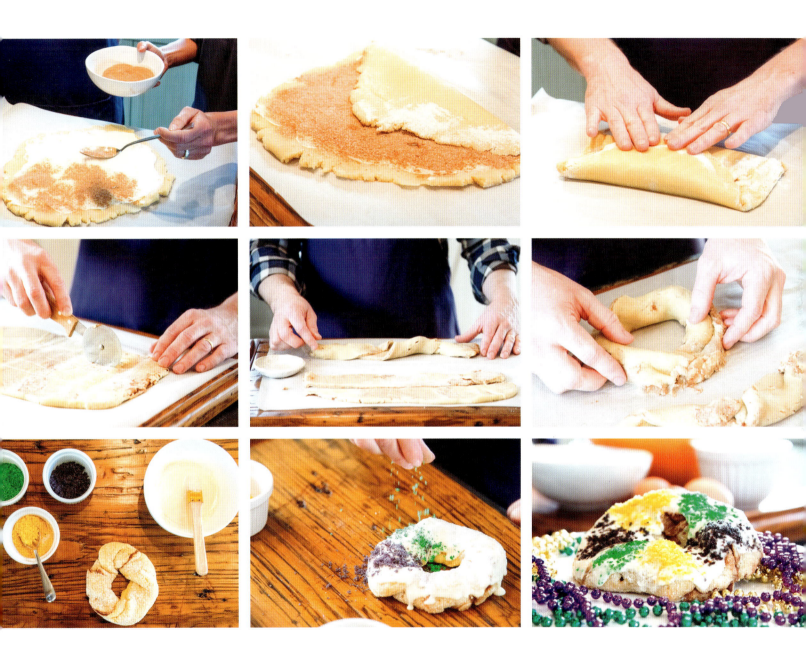

## Tip/

For those new to gluten-free baking, it can be helpful to stick with tried and true recipes for a while, to get a feel for what works and what doesn't.

# Gluten Free Flours 101

Gluten is a protein found in wheat, rye, and barley that gives dough its elasticity and helps bread to rise, giving texture, structure, and shape to baked goods. Many gluten-free flours are better for us, especially when they're lower in carbs, higher in protein, fiber, and heart-smart fats and have a lower glycemic index. But buying gluten-free flours is one thing; knowing how to cook and bake with these flours can be the challenge.

Baking with gluten-free flours requires additional ingredients that make up for the lack of gluten, like xanthan gum or whey protein powder, to help with structure and allow baked goods to rise. Here's the rundown on two of our favorite gluten free flours.

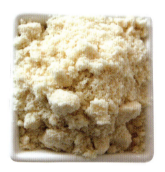

**ALMOND FLOUR** Low carb, high fat, high moisture.

Use **MORE ALMOND FLOUR** than the amount of wheat flour that the original recipe calls for—up to 50% more.

Use less liquid: cut back on liquid by as much as 50%.

Almond flour can be used for breading meats and vegetables.

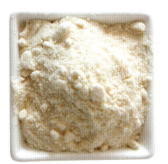

**COCONUT FLOUR** Low carb, high fiber, low moisture.

Use **LESS COCONUT FLOUR** than the amount of wheat flour that the original recipe calls for—as much as 50% less.

Use more liquids: typically an equal ratio of liquid to coconut flour.

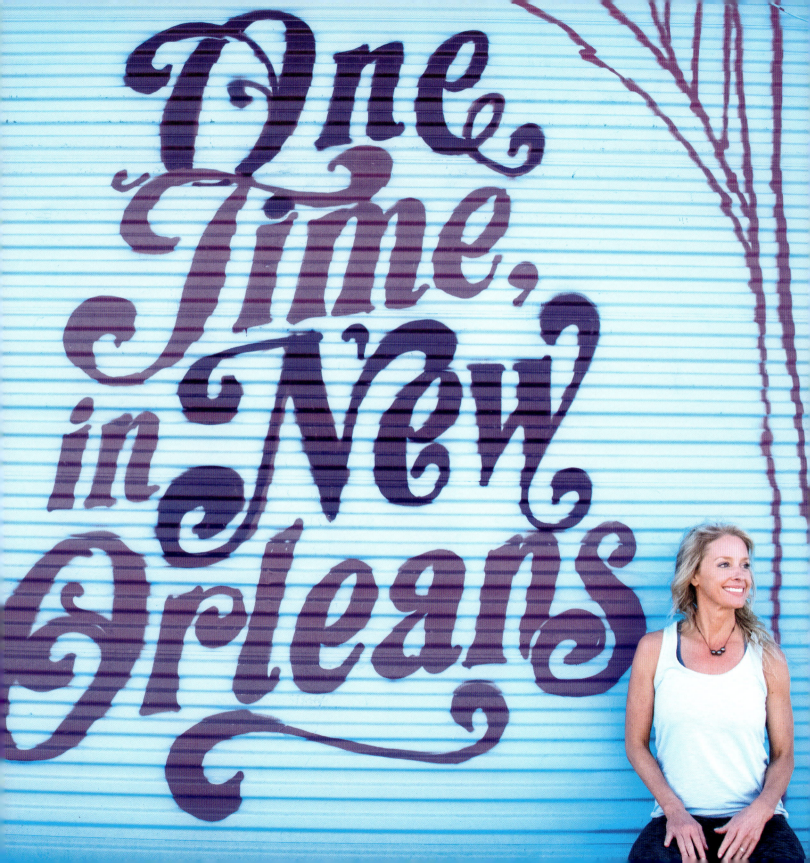

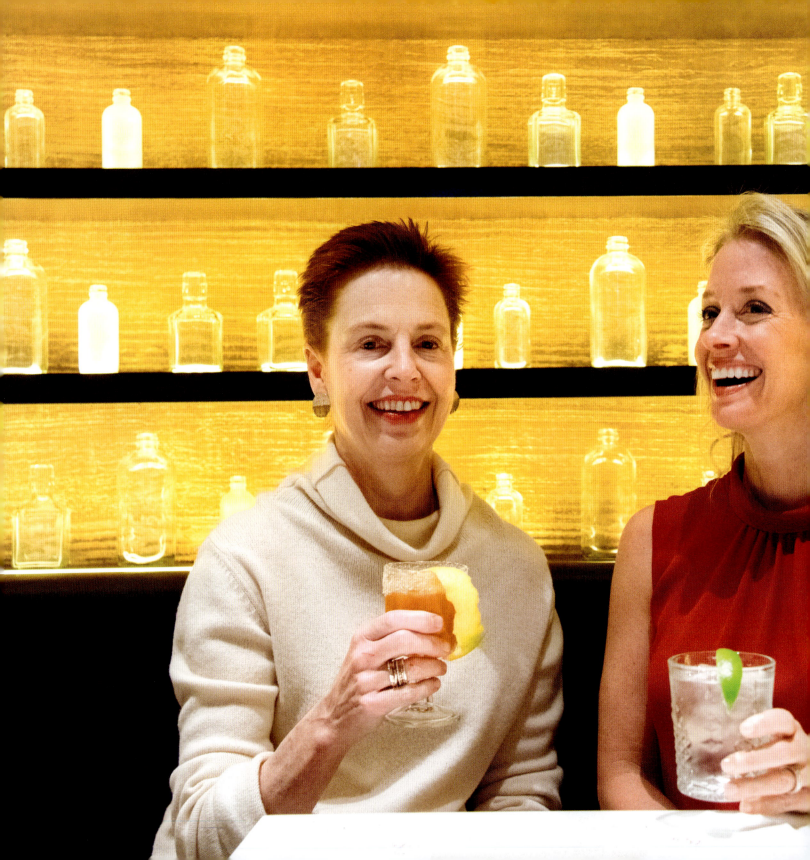

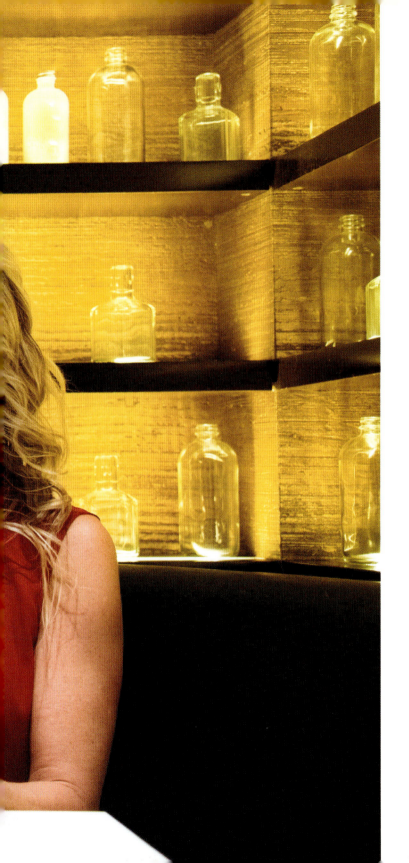

# 8
# SIP

## Cocktails, Zero Proof Cocktails + Refreshers

"A great meal starts with a great cocktail!"
—Ti Martin of Commander's Palace

We agree with Ti, and because every night may not be "cocktail worthy," our Eat Fit bartenders, chefs, and mixologists have created a solid repertoire of drinks to suit every occasion.

It's no secret that in the South we love food, we love parties, we love festivals, we love family, and we love to drink. For many, dialing back on alcohol can be even more challenging than changing how we eat. Our Sips start out as zero proof cocktails; each can easily be transformed into a full-proof cocktail. But with drinks like these, you may not even miss the booze.

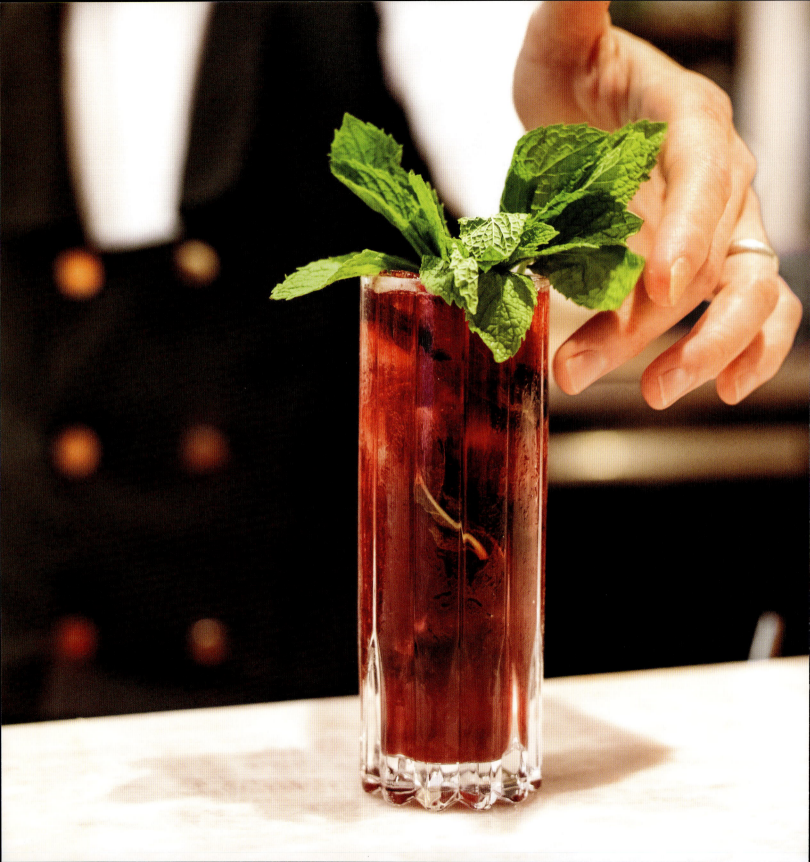

# Hibiscus Blackberry Cooler
## *Miss River*

**Makes 4 servings**

A perfect porch sipper. Native to the wetlands of Louisiana, the flowers, leaves, and seeds of the hibiscus plant are all edible. And beyond its beautiful hue and vibrant flavor, hibiscus tea has been shown to benefit blood pressure. Hibiscus tea can be steeped from loose leaf tea or tea bags; enjoy it hot or cold, and steep an extra batch to keep on hand for flavor-infused hydration.

**2 cups hibiscus tea (loose leaf or bagged), steeped**
**1 cup fresh mint leaves**
**1 tablespoon stevia sweetener (or plant-based sweetener of choice)**
**1 lime, juiced (approximately 2 tablespoons lime juice)**
**12-ounce bottle or can of sparkling water**
**8 blackberries**

Steep tea according to directions. Wash mint and set aside half for later. Place remaining mint leaves and stevia in a large glass jar and use a wooden spoon to muddle. Pour hibiscus tea over mint leaves, cover, and refrigerate for at least 3 hours.

Once chilled, strain the tea with a fine mesh sieve. Add lime juice and stir. Add more sweetener if preferred.

To serve, smash a few mint leaves and a blackberry at the bottom of a tall Collins glass. Fill glass with ice, add 3 ounces of hibiscus mint blend, and stir. Top with three ounces of sparkling water. Garnish with a blackberry and mint sprig.

**PER SERVING:** 10 calories, 0 fat, 0 saturated fat, 15 mg sodium, 2 grams carbohydrate (2 grams net carbs), 0 fiber, <1 gram sugar (0 added sugar), 0 protein
**GF, Low Carb, Vegan, Low Sodium**

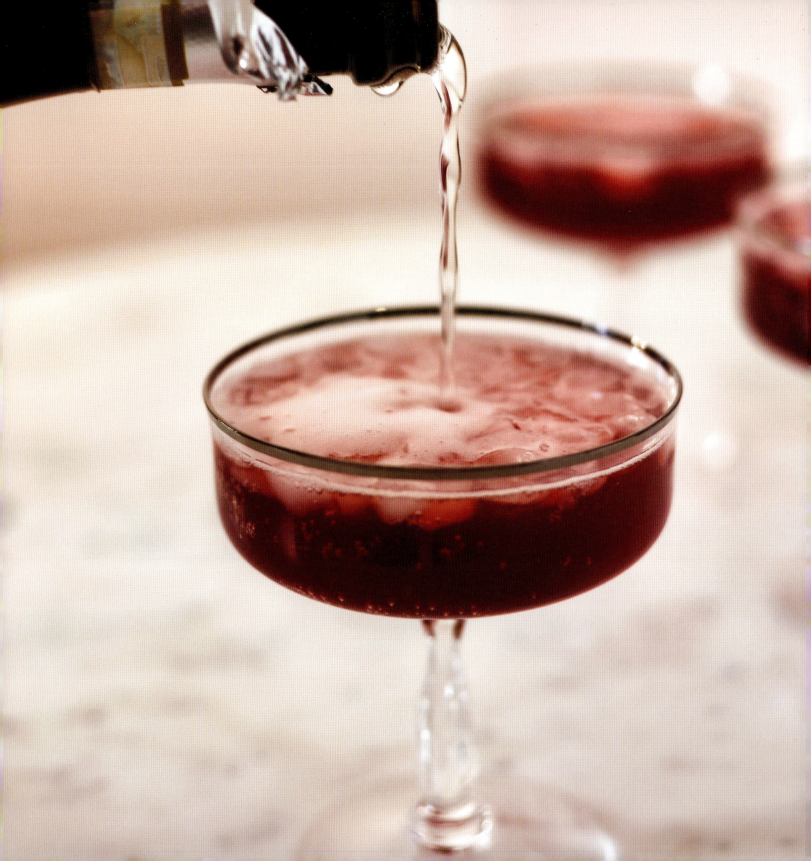

# Cherry Sparkle
## Eat Fit Collection

**Makes 4 servings**

A "shrub" is a vintage syrup-style mixer that lends a refreshing complexity and sweet tartness that elevates a cocktail. Typically centered on sugar and vinegar, our Eat Fit version is made with a plant-based sweetener and apple cider vinegar, both naturally stabilizing for our energy and insulin levels. But health benefits aside, this zero proof cocktail brings flavor and beauty, effortlessly.

1 cup cherries, pitted (fresh cherries, or frozen and thawed)
1 cup Swerve Granular
1½ cups water
3 ounces apple cider vinegar
Sparkling water or zero proof sparkling wine, for serving

To make the cherry shrub, add cherries, Swerve Granular, and water to a medium saucepan over low heat, stirring occasionally until cherries are very soft, approximately 10-15 minutes. Pour mixture through a sieve and return to the saucepan. Add vinegar and return heat to medium-low, bringing it to a slow boil. Remove from heat, transfer to a heat-safe container such as a mason jar, and let cool.

To serve, add approximately 1½ ounces of the cherry shrub to a coupe glass. Top with a splash of sparkling water or zero proof sparkling wine and serve.

**PER SERVING (WITH SPARKLING WATER):** 5 calories, 0 fat, 0 saturated fat, 0 sodium, <1 gram carbohydrate, 0 fiber, <1 gram sugar (0 added sugar), 0 protein
GF, Low Carb, Vegan, Low Sodium

## Save for Later/

Refrigerate any remaining shrub syrup in a sealed glass container for up to one week.

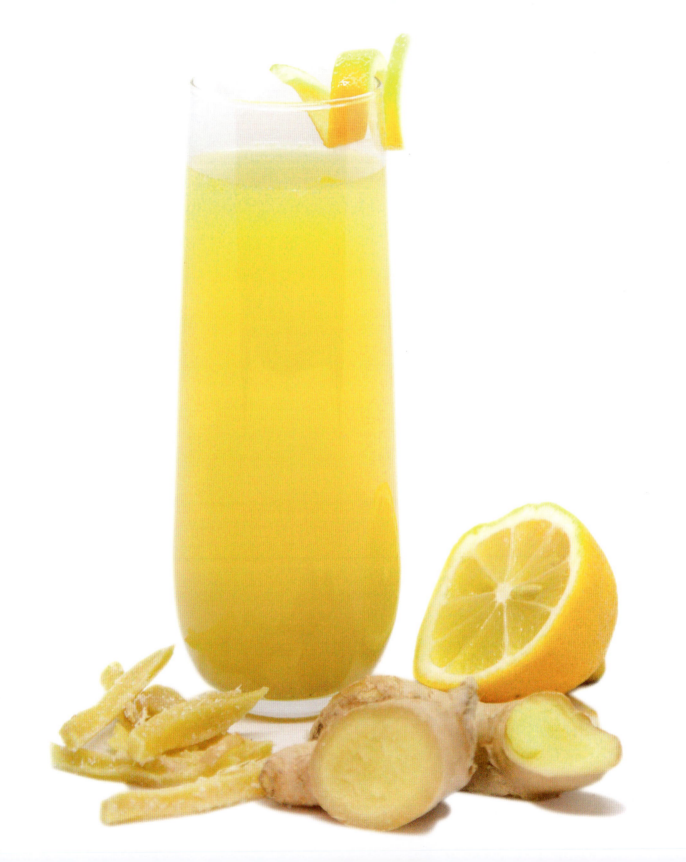

# Candied Ginger Lemon Drop
## *Eat Fit Collection*

**Makes 4 servings**

This booze-free toddy goes down like a smooth bourbon but keeps you walking a straight line all night.

- 3 inches ginger root, peeled and sliced
- ¾ cup Swerve Granular (2 tablespoons reserved)
- 1½ cups water
- ½ cup fresh lemon juice
- 1 liter chilled club soda
- Lemon peel, for garnish

In a saucepan over medium heat, combine ginger slices, Swerve (all but reserved 2 tablespoons), and water. Stir until Swerve dissolves. Boil for about 20 minutes, until syrup begins to thicken. Remove from heat, strain to remove ginger, and let cool. Toss ginger slices with reserved Swerve to coat and set aside.

In a pitcher or cocktail shaker with ice, combine ginger syrup and lemon juice. Stir or shake to mix. Divide amongst 4 glasses, fill each to rim with club soda, and garnish with a slice of candied ginger and a twirl of lemon peel.

**PER SERVING:** 15 calories, 0 fat, 0 saturated fat, 55 mg sodium, 39 grams carbohydrate (<1 gram net carb), 2 grams fiber, 2 grams sugar (0 added sugar), 0 protein

GF, Low Carb, Vegan, Low Sodium

## Make It a Cocktail

Add 1½ ounces of bourbon to each drink.

## Love It Later

Make an extra batch or two of the candied ginger for snacking. You'll thank us later.

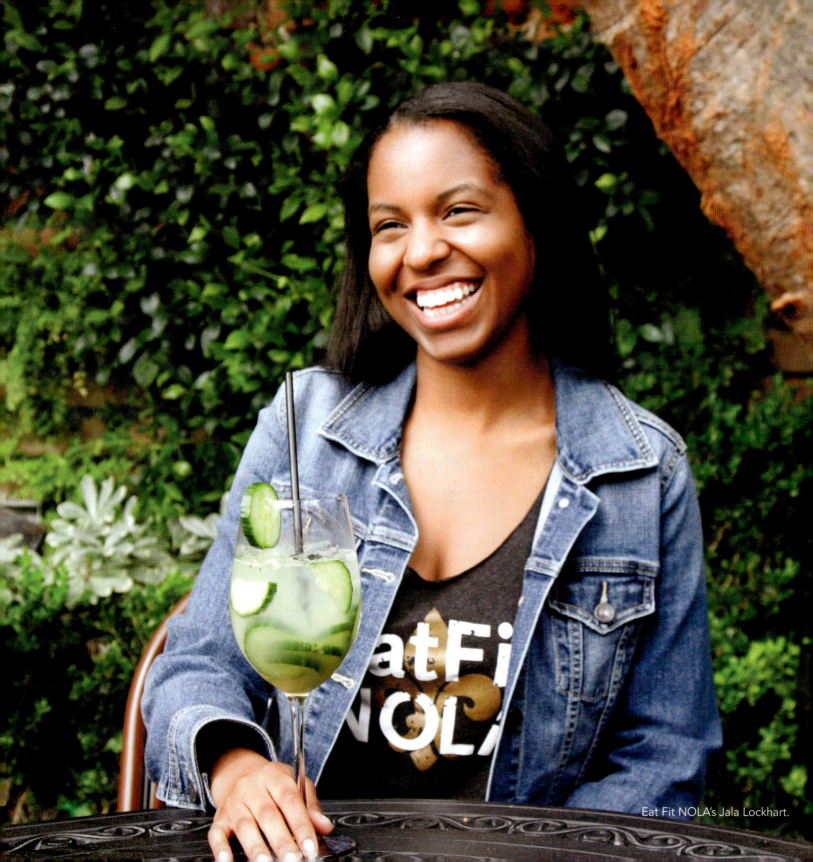

Eat Fit NOLA's Jala Lockhart.

# Cucumber-Lime Mojito
## Don Juanz Baja Beach Tacos

**Makes 2 servings**

Don Juanz was one of our first Eat Fit Shreveport partners – plus, they always bring the party – so we love that we get to showcase this fun—and easy-peasy— zero proof mojito as part of our Eat Fit Shreveport line-up.

**4 cucumber slices**
**1 lime cut into 6 half-wheels, divided**
**1 ounce Eat Fit Simple Syrup (recipe follows)**
**10 ounces club soda, divided**

Muddle cucumber and 4 lime wheels in a cocktail shaker. Add Eat Fit Simple Syrup and club soda. Shake to mix. Spoon the muddled mixture into 2 glasses. Fill with ice then top with any remaining club soda. Garnish with remaining lime and serve.

**PER SERVING:** 15 calories, 0 fat, 0 saturated fat, 30 mg sodium, 11 grams carbohydrate (4 grams net carbs), 1 gram fiber, 1 gram sugar (0 added sugar), 0 protein

GF, Low Carb, Vegan, Low Sodium

## Make It a Cocktail/

Add 1½ ounces of clear rum to each drink.

## Ingredient Improv/

Don't stop with cucumber. Muddle any type of fruits, herbs (think basil, rosemary, cilantro), spices (we love adding ginger, cinnamon, or cayenne), even jalapeño. The combinations are endless.

# Eat Fit Simple Syrup
## The Eat Fit Collection

**Makes ½ cup**

Swerve and allulose both can work for simple syrup, but we prefer allulose since it won't recrystallize or settle out.

**½ cup water**
**½ cup Swerve Granular or 1 ½ cups granular allulose**

In a saucepan, bring water to a boil. Reduce to medium-high heat and add sweetener. Stir to dissolve and continue to heat for 10 minutes. Pour into heat-safe glass container and refrigerate to chill. Store unused portion in an airtight container in a refrigerator for up to 4 weeks.

**PER TWO TABLESPOONS:** 0 calories, 0 fat, 0 saturated fat, 0 sodium, 0 carbohydrates, 0 fiber, 0 sugar, 0 protein

GF, Low Carb, Vegan, Low Sodium

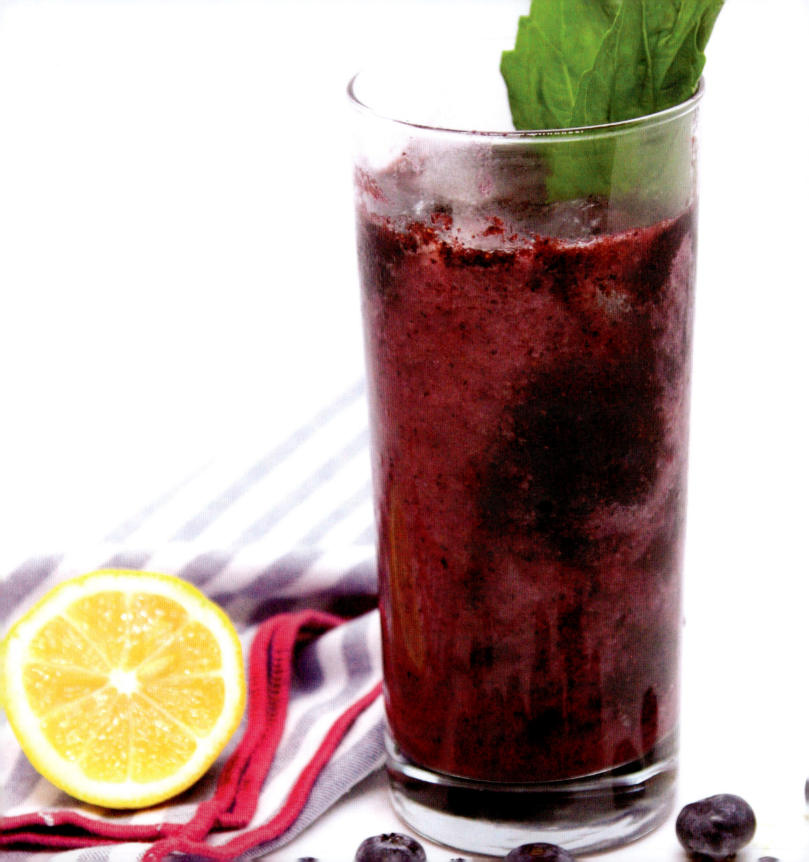

# Blueberry Basil Lemonade
## Eat Fit Collection

**Makes 6 servings**

Bursting with the flavors of summer, our refreshing, colorful, and citrusy Blueberry Basil Lemonade is a perfect poolside treat.

**For the Basil Simple Syrup**
½ packed cup torn fresh basil leaves
¾ cup Swerve Granular
⅔ cup water

**For the Blueberry Lemonade**
2 cups blueberries (fresh or frozen)
½ cup basil simple syrup
¾ cup lemon juice, freshly squeezed
1 tablespoon lemon zest

**For the Blueberry Puree**
1 cup blueberries
¼ cup Swerve Granular

**For the Garnish**
Lemon slices
Fresh blueberries
Basil sprigs

**Make the Basil Simple Syrup:** In a saucepan over medium heat, combine basil, Swerve, and water. Stir until Swerve dissolves. Boil for 5 minutes then remove from heat, leaving the basil leaves to steep for 10 minutes. Strain to remove the basil, pressing on the leaves to get every last bit of herbal goodness. Refrigerate until ready to use.

**Make the Blueberry Lemonade:** Combine blueberries, basil simple syrup, lemon juice, and lemon zest in a blender. Puree until very smooth. Strain with a fine mesh sieve and set aside.

**Prepare the Blueberry Puree:** Blend blueberries and Swerve until pureed.

Fill glasses with ice and add 1 tablespoon of blueberry puree to each. Top with blueberry lemonade. Garnish with lemon slices, blueberries, and a sprig of basil.

**PER SERVING:** 50 calories, 0 fat, 0 saturated fat, 0 sodium, 30 grams carbohydrate (11 grams net carbs), 3 grams fiber, 9 grams sugar (0 added sugar), <1 gram protein
GF, Vegan, Low Sodium

## Make It a Cocktail

Add 1½ ounces of vodka to each drink.

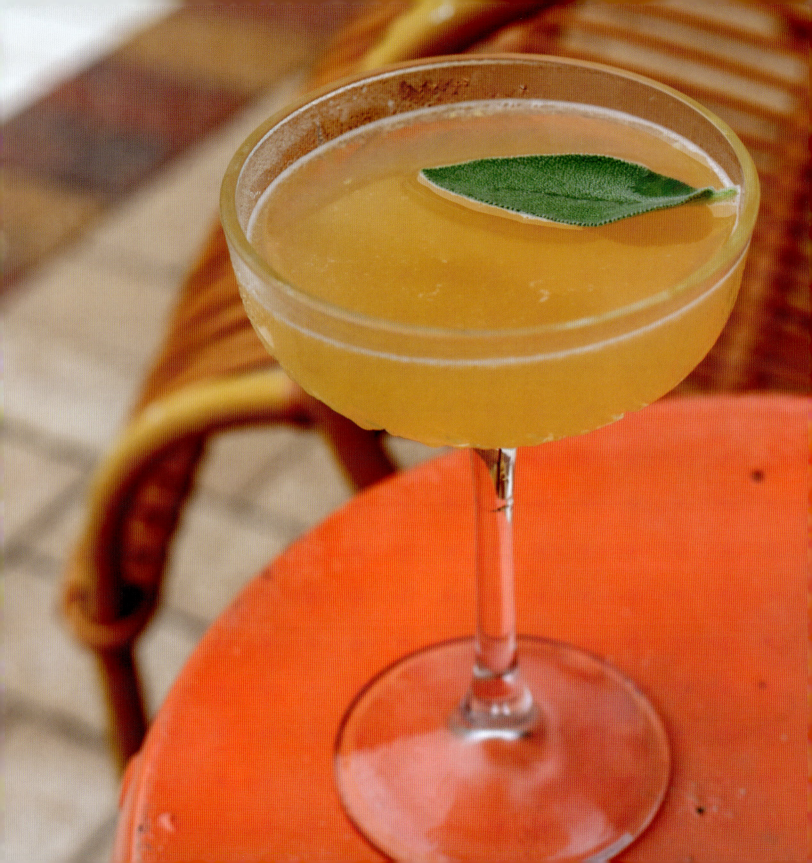

# Sage Advice
## Cypress Bar at The Southern Hotel

**Makes 2 servings**

Created by Christopher Walker, bar manager of the Cypress Bar at the Southern Hotel, this award-winning zero proof cocktail is elegantly refreshing. Chris created this Eat Fit version for us with a natural, no-sugar Elderflower Syrup to complement the grapefruit and sage.

**2 ounces fresh grapefruit juice**
**3 tablespoons lemon juice**
**2 tablespoons Elderflower Syrup (recipe follows)**
**4 sage leaves**
**Ice**
**6 ounces sparkling water**

Place grapefruit juice, lemon juice, Elderflower Syrup, and 2 sage leaves with ice in shaker. Shake thoroughly and double strain into two chilled coupe glasses. Top with sparkling water and expressed sage leaf. Slap or smack sage leaves first to fully release their aromatics before garnishing.

PER SERVING: 20 calories, 0 fat, 0 saturated fat, 0 sodium, 5 grams carbohydrates (5 net carbs), 0 fiber, <1 gram sugar (0 added sugar), 0 protein
GF, Low Carb, Vegan, Low Sodium

ELDERFLOWER SYRUP
**15 fresh or dried elderflowers**
**1 batch Eat Fit Simple Syrup (page 225)**

In a saucepan over low heat, add 15 elderflower heads (flowers only, no stems) to a batch of Eat Fit Simple Syrup. Stir and heat for 10 minutes. Transfer to a heat-safe glass container and allow to infuse for at least 1 hour. Strain before using; refrigerate for up to 4 weeks.

PER SERVING: 0 calories, 0 fat, 0 saturated fat, 0 sodium, 0 carbohydrates, 0 fiber, 0 sugar, 0 protein
GF, Low Carb, Vegan, Low Sodium

## Elderflowers

Elderflowers can be purchased online, and it's also surprisingly easy to grow our own. A perennial that requires little effort to grow, the elder bush gives us beauty and berries, as well as flowers.

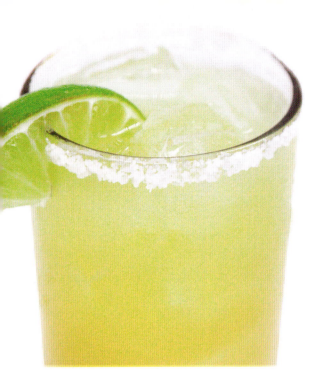

# Superior Margarita
## Superior Grill

**Makes 2 servings**

There is no reason to take things to a whole 'nother level with this margarita recipe. It is so delicious, it's easy to overlook that it's also alcohol free.

**4 ounces orange juice**
**¼ cup lime juice**
**2 tablespoons Swerve Confectioners**
**6-8 ounces club soda**
**Lime wheel, for garnish**

Combine orange juice, lime juice, and Swerve in a cocktail shaker with ice. Shake and strain into a Collins glass filled with ice. Top with club soda and garnish with lime.

PER SERVING: 35 calories, 0 fat, 0 saturated fat, 35 mg sodium, 15 grams carbohydrate (9 grams net carbs), 0 fiber, 5 grams sugar (0 added sugar), 0 protein
GF, Low Carb, Vegan, Low Sodium

## Make It a Cocktail

Add 1½ ounces of tequila to each drink.

# Fire Tonic Virgin Mary
## Andi Lynn's Pure & Custom Formulary

**Makes 2 servings**

In south Louisiana, the Bloody Mary is a quintessential brunch or game-day cocktail, usually adorned with enough vegetables to make us feel like we're having a salad. This "Virgin Mary" is equally substantial but lower sodium and sans the alcohol. And for those who want to keep things chill even while friends are stepping it up, a Virgin Mary looks just like the real thing. No one even questions if you're drinking.

¼ cup Andi Lynn's Fire Raw Apple Cider Tonic
12 ounces low-sodium tomato juice
2 teaspoons Tabasco
½ teaspoon Lea & Perrins Worcestershire sauce
2 tablespoons horseradish
1 lime, juiced
Dash of black pepper
Lime or lemon wedge, for garnish
Slices of yellow peppers, for garnish
Fresh herbs, for garnish

Combine all ingredients except garnish in a glass or cocktail mixer with a handful of ice cubes. Shake or stir to mix. Garnish with lime or lemon wedge, peppers, and fresh herbs.

PER SERVING: 50 calories, 0 fat, 0 saturated fat, 210 mg sodium, 12 grams carbohydrate (10 grams net carbs), 2 grams fiber, 7 grams sugar (0 added sugar), 1 gram protein
GF

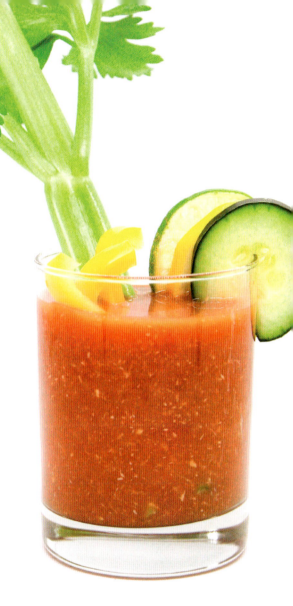

## Make It a Cocktail

Add 1½ ounces of vodka to each drink.

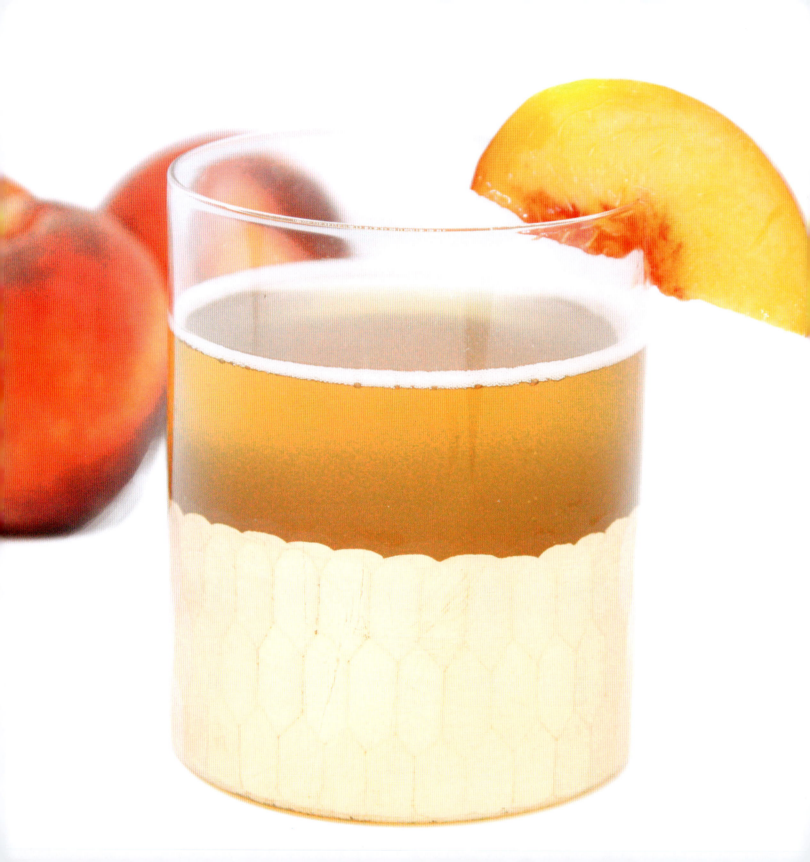

# Bucha Bellini
## *Big Easy Bucha*

**Makes 2 servings**

Who doesn't love a Bellini? This delightfully peachy drink is a perfect choice for (put your wine down) Wednesday.

**16 ounces Big Easy Bucha Front Porch Peach kombucha (or any sweet, floral variety of kombucha)**
**2 tablespoons El Guapo Summer Berries Bitters (or any citrus or berry-based bitters)**
**Peach slices, for garnish**

Pour and garnish. It's that simple.

PER SERVING: 30 calories, 0 fat, 0 saturated fat, 10 mg sodium, 7 grams carbohydrate (7 grams net carbs), 0 fiber, 2 grams sugar, 0 protein
GF, Low Carb, Vegetarian, Low Sodium

## Make It a Cocktail /

Go halfsies: Fill a champagne flute with half peach kombucha and half Prosecco, champagne, or sparkling wine, and garnish with slice of peach.

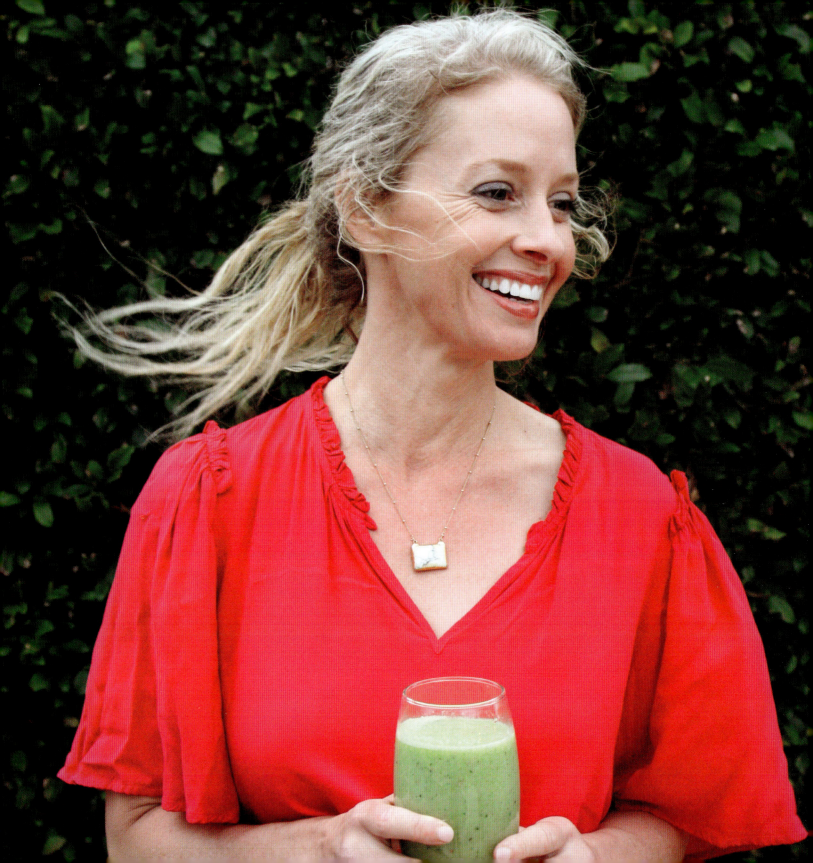

# Green Goddess Smoothie
## FUEL Café + Market at Ochsner Fitness Center

**Makes 2 servings**

This smoothie immediately makes us feel all glowy and energized.

2 cups water
2 scoops collagen powder (e.g. hydrolyzed collagen or collagen peptides)
½ avocado
2 cups fresh spinach
1 cup chopped cucumber with peel
2 tablespoons diced celery
½ cup frozen apple slices
1 medium banana
3 leaves fresh basil
2 tablespoons lemon juice
Cucumber slices, for garnish

Combine all ingredients in a blender and blend until smooth.

**PER SERVING:** 240 calories, 8 grams fat, 1 gram saturated fat, 150 mg sodium, 26 grams carbohydrate (19 grams net carbs), 7 grams fiber, 12 grams sugar (0 added sugar), 23 grams protein
**GF**

## Why Collagen /

**Joint health:** May boost the health of ligaments and tendons, helping to improve joint health and joint pain.

**Healthy hair, skin, and nails:** Supports the density and structure of the body's collagen and helps reduce collagen breakdown, in turn improving skin elasticity and hydration.

**GI health:** Helps to heal and protect the lining of the GI tract, improving nutrient absorption and digestion.

**More fullness, improved weight management:** The amino acids in collagen help to keep us feeling fuller longer. Adding a scoop or two of collagen to your morning latte or afternoon smoothie can help to keep your appetite in check for hours.

## Make It Vegan /

Replace the collagen with vanilla plant-based protein powder.

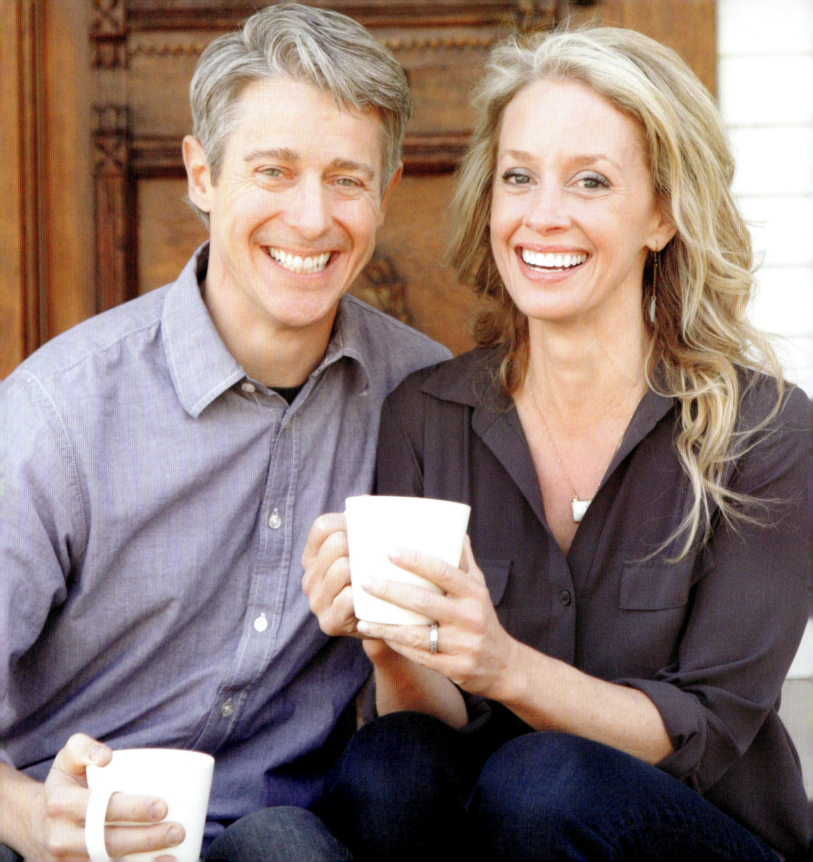

# Collagen Café Frappe
## FUEL Café + Market at Ochsner Fitness Center

**Makes 2 servings**

This is my go-to afternoon pick-me-up. It's like one of those frozen blended coffee drinks that are crazy-high in sugar, but this recipe has zero added sugar, a hefty dose of collagen, and the protein equivalent of approximately 4 ounces of lean meat.

12 ounces unsweetened vanilla almond milk
6 ounces chilled coffee concentrate
2 scoops vanilla protein powder (whey or plant protein)
2 scoops collagen powder (e.g. hydrolyzed collagen or collagen peptides)
2 teaspoons Swerve Granular
1 heaping scoop ice

Combine all ingredients in a blender and blend until smooth.

PER SERVING: 160 calories, 4 grams fat, 1 gram saturated fat, 260 mg sodium, 7 grams carbohydrate (3 grams net carbs), <1 gram fiber, 2 grams sugar (0 added sugar), 30 grams protein
GF, Low Carb

Brad and Molly

## Protein Powder 101

**Whey Protein:** Easily digested and absorbed, making it a great pre- and post-workout option for fueling and recovery.

**Plant-Based Vegan Protein Powders:** Typically centered on pea protein, hemp, brown rice, and quinoa, these protein powders are a good option for those looking to avoid dairy or soy.

**Casein:** A slow-digesting protein, resulting in a slow release of amino acids. I typically recommend casein before bedtime to minimize overnight muscle loss, but it can be useful throughout the day for those looking to feel fuller longer.

# Index

**A**

| | |
|---|---|
| Artisan Berry Cheesecake | 201 |
| Attiki Chicken Shawarma Marinade | 135 |
| Avocado Puree | 114 |
| Avocado Salad | 91 |

**B**

| | |
|---|---|
| Baba Ganoush | 41 |
| Baingan Bharta | 63 |
| Balsamic Reduction | 33 |
| Beet Hummus | 45 |
| Beet Medallions | 164 |
| Blueberry Basil Lemonade | 227 |
| Blueberry Beet Barbecue Sauce | 185 |
| Blueberry Protein Muffin | 203 |
| Braised Lamb Shank with Pomegranate Glaze and Labneh | 129 |
| Brown Curry Powder | 61 |
| Brussels + Broccoli Mash | 155 |
| Brutti Ma Buoni | 197 |
| Bucha Bellini | 233 |
| Butternut Squash Hash | 158 |

**C**

| | |
|---|---|
| Candied Ginger Lemon Drop | 223 |
| Candied Walnuts | 167 |
| Caramelized Sweet Potato with Labneh and Chimichurri | 39 |
| Carrot Hummus | 43 |
| Cauliflower Nachos | 37 |
| Cedar Plank Smoked Salmon | 31 |
| Charred Cabbage with Hazelnut Muhammara and Tahini | 153 |
| Cherry Sparkle | 221 |
| Chicken Shawarma Lettuce Cups | 135 |
| Chimichurri | 184 |
| Chipotle Crema | 184 |
| Chocolate Chip Cookies | 195 |
| Chopped Mediterranean Salad | 93 |
| Cleo's House Seasoning Blend | 91 |
| Cleo's Lemon Dressing | 172 |
| Coconut Brown Rice | 60 |
| Coconut Milk Curry | 133 |
| Coffee Cured Duck Breast Salad with Quinoa + Kale | 127 |
| Collagen Café Frappe | 237 |
| Confit Garlic + Garlic Oil | 45 |
| Crabmeat + Artichoke Salad with Citrus Dressing | 81 |
| Crawfish Boil Quiche | 123 |
| Crawfish Mushroom + Goat Cheese Bisque | 67 |
| Creole Lemon Vinaigrette | 176 |
| Cucumber-Lime Mojito | 225 |
| Cured. House Seasoning Blend | 45 |
| Curried Carrot + Coconut Soup with Jumbo Lump Crab + Lime | 55 |

**D**

| | |
|---|---|
| Day-Brightening Curry Chicken Salad | 137 |
| Demi-Glace | 143 |

**E**

| | |
|---|---|
| Eat Fit Berry Reduction | 186 |
| Eat Fit Simple Syrup | 225 |
| Eggplant Croutons | 165 |
| Elderflower Syrup | 229 |
| Esmeralda Dressing | 89 |
| Esmeralda Salad | 89 |

**F**

| | |
|---|---|
| Field Pea Curry | 60 |
| Fig Street Fig Salad | 83 |
| Fire Tonic Virgin Mary | 231 |
| Fresh Basil Vinaigrette | 172 |
| Frutti di Mare Portofino | 125 |

**G**

| | |
|---|---|
| Ginger Dressing | 171 |
| Ginger Garlic Paste | 63 |
| Ginger Pickled Mirliton | 163 |
| Green Chili Glaze | 102 |
| Green Chili Glazed Grilled Salmon | 101 |
| Green Curry Base | 53 |
| Green Goddess Smoothie | 235 |
| Griddled Summer Squash and Tender Greens | 90 |
| Grilled Fish + Shrimp with Corn Maque Choux + Creole Lemon Vinaigrette | 111 |
| Grilled Garlic Shrimp with White Beans + Pickled Okra Giardiniera | 119 |
| Grilled Pork Tenderloin with Blueberry Beet Barbeque Sauce | 141 |
| Grilled Shrimp with Black Bean Cake + Avocado Puree | 113 |
| Grilled Steak Salad with Red Wine Vinaigrette | 145 |
| Guacamole | 28 |

**H**

| | |
|---|---|
| Harissa Paste | 133 |
| Harissa Spiced Lamb Loin in Coconut Milk Curry + Quinoa | 132 |
| Hibiscus Blackberry Cooler | 219 |

**I**

| | |
|---|---|
| Insalate Caprese | 35 |

## J
| | |
|---|---|
| Jacques-Imo's Citrus Dressing | 81 |
| Jicama Slaw | 95 |
| Jumbo Lump Crab + Lime Topping | 56 |
| Jumbo Lump Crab Cakes | 17 |

## L
| | |
|---|---|
| Labneh | 174 |
| Lemon Scones | 209 |

## M
| | |
|---|---|
| Mango Chutney | 186 |
| Mango Tuna Sashimi Salad | 147 |
| Maple Pecan Butter | 187 |
| Matbucha | 175 |
| Mediterranean Whole Lentil Soup | 77 |
| Minted Pea Puree | 102 |
| Mirliton Salad | 102 |
| Miso Vinaigrette | 171 |
| Muhammara | 174 |
| Mushroom Stock | 68 |

## O
| | |
|---|---|
| Orleans Sauce | 109 |

## P
| | |
|---|---|
| Peach Pie with Whipped Goat Cheese | 199 |
| Pear and Ricotta Tartine with Maple Pecan Butter | 33 |
| Petite Cartwright Filet | 143 |
| Pickled Okra Giardiniera | 119 |
| Pickled Red Onions | 163 |
| Pompano en Papillote | 105 |
| Ponzu Sauce | 28 |
| Poppyseed Berry Vinaigrette | 177 |

## Q
| | |
|---|---|
| Quinoa | 132 |

## R
| | |
|---|---|
| Raspberry Mint Vinaigrette | 177 |
| Ravigote Sauce | 183 |
| Red Beans + Cauliflower Rice | 65 |
| Red Wine Vinaigrette | 178 |
| Redfish Orleans | 109 |
| Remoulade Sauce | 181 |
| Rice Wine Vinaigrette | 28 |
| Roasted Mushrooms | 164 |
| Roasted Pepper Quinoa Pilaf | 159 |
| Rosemary Garlic Biscuits | 205 |
| Rustic Eat Fit King Cake | 211 |

## S
| | |
|---|---|
| Sage Advice | 229 |
| Salted Dark Chocolate Peanut Butter Cups | 193 |
| Sambal Vegetable Stir Fry | 166 |
| Sautéed Swiss Chard | 157 |
| Scampi-Style Shrimp + Creamy Cauliflower Grits | 75 |
| Seafood Cioppino | 71 |
| Seafood Tomato Stock | 71 |
| Shrimp + Mirliton Stuffed Peppers | 117 |
| Shrimp Mosca | 121 |
| Shrimp Quinoa Jambalaya | 73 |
| Shrimp Remoulade | 19 |
| Shrimp Salad with Raspberry Mint Vinaigrette | 21 |
| Smoked Tomato Basil Soup | 51 |
| Steen's Cane Vinaigrette | 179 |
| Strawberry Fields Forever with Tea-Infused Berry Vinaigrette | 87 |
| Summer Melon Salad | 85 |
| Superior Margarita | 230 |
| Sweet Corn Creole Cream Cheese | 141 |
| Sweet Potato Carnival Soup | 49 |
| Sweet Potato Snapper | 99 |

## T
| | |
|---|---|
| Tahini | 173 |
| Tea-Infused Berry Vinaigrette | 178 |
| Thai Chicken Marinade | 139 |
| Thai Green Curry | 53 |
| Thai Peanut Dressing | 176 |
| Thai Quinoa + Kale Salad with Grilled Chicken | 139 |
| Tofu + Eggplant in Field Pea Curry | 59 |

## V
| | |
|---|---|
| Vietnamese-Style Crawfish Canapé on Spiced Cucumber Medallions | 23 |

## W
| | |
|---|---|
| White Beans | 161 |
| Wilted Kale + Roasted Cauliflower "Risotto" | 151 |

## Y
| | |
|---|---|
| Yellowfin Tuna Poke Tostada | 27 |